Epilepsy Explained

A book for people who want to know more about epilepsy

Ulrich Altrup
Professor of Experimental Epileptology
University of Münster
Germany

Christian E. Elger
Professor of Epileptology
University of Bonn
Germany

Markus Reuber
Senior Lecturer in Neurology
University of Sheffield
United Kingdom

Medicine Explained Publishing Lienen

Published 2005 by
Medicine Explained Publishing
Muehlenweg 7, 49536 Lienen, Germany
ISBN 3-9809638-1-0

Printed by: QuickPrinter, Overath

Epilepsy Explained

A book for people who want to know more about epilepsy

Epilepsy, a problem with the brain
Recognising epilepsy
Treating epilepsy
Epilepsy in everyday life

Medicine Explained Publishing   Lienen

Foreword

Epilepsy has been the topic of countless books. Indeed the present authors remind us that there is a mention in the "Codex Hammurabi", the world's oldest known book. So why another and what makes this one different? The first clue is in the title, *Epilepsy Explained*, and the second lies in the comment on page six, "It [this book] was written to inform people about epilepsy. It is meant to be understood by everyone."

Many text books are dry and full of facts and statistics. They may seek to explain their subject, but all too often the reader has to work hard to understand them. In *Epilepsy Explained*, Ulrich Altrup, Christian E. Elger and Markus Reuber go far beyond that and truly explain the mysteries of epilepsy to the reader. Moreover, they do it in a style that is easy on the mind but not patronising. This book will be equally at home with the ordinary person and on the professional's shelf as a reference when explaining epilepsy to a patient.

The structure and function of the brain is described in detail and in language accessible by anyone. Alongside this description is a considerable number of clear and simple but informative diagrams. At the same time, the book is challenging. So there are activities for the reader to undertake, such as 'find out how many people in your community have epilepsy.' The book does not shy away from the difficult topics either. It tackles sudden unexpected death in epilepsy and, from a technical viewpoint, describes in clear detail modern diagnostic tools such as CT and MRI scanning.

The book is not only clear but also comprehensive, covering topics from first aid during seizures, through treatment and everyday life to medications, the law and prejudice. It is refreshing to see prejudice tackled, especially as quality of life issues have become such an important part of managing epilepsy. Useful information includes how to use alcohol sensibly, how to assess the risk in sports and how to plan travel.

Nothing is perfect though and I have a few minor criticisms. The doctor may well view absence epilepsy as mild. As an educator and knowing how often absence seizures are missed in the assessment of children, I would not necessarily view these as mild. However this criticism must not detract from the quality of this book, its content and the refreshing presentation of such an important subject. *Epilepsy Explained* deserves a wide readership.

Ronald Radley
Chairman, Epilepsy Action
Former Headteacher, school for children with epilepsy

Author's Foreword

Epilepsy is one of the commonest disorders of the brain not often discussed in the open. The fears and prejudice associated with the condition can make life harder for people with epilepsy than it needs to be. In this book, the authors want to provide information about all aspects of epilepsy. The book has been written for people with epilepsy, but also for their families, friends, teachers, and carers.

For this English edition, the book has been extended and thoroughly updated. Ten years ago this book started as a set of posters entitled "Epilepsy, a common problem", which were shown during an open week at an epilepsy centre in Germany. The authors sometimes had to simplify complicated subject areas. In striking a balance between scientific accuracy and a more accessible presentation, we felt that it was more important that our explanations were easy to understand. Many people have helped us with this book. We are especially grateful to Dr. A. Hecker, Dr. M. Finzel, Dr. J. von Oertzen, Dr. S. Ried, Dr. U. Specht, Prof. E.-J. Speckmann, and Prof. P. Wolf. We would like to thank D. Cockman as well as S. Wagstaff and M. Cooper from Epilepsy Action for helping to edit the manuscript. This book could not have been published without the support of S. Wigglesworth, R. Radley and Dr. J. Bird of Epilepsy Action and an educational grant from Pfizer Incorporated. The drawings of people with epilepsy and their seizures were produced by L. Vollmert and G. Jakobs (supported by Prof. M. Herrenberger) from the Department of Design at the Polytechnical University of Münster, Germany.

Münster, Bonn, Sheffield
September 2004

Ulrich Altrup
Christian E. Elger
Markus Reuber

Contents in brief

Content in detail

1 Epilepsy, a problem with the brain

2 Recognising epilepsy

3 Treating epilepsy

4. Epilepsy in everyday life

1 Epilepsy, a problem with the brain

Summary

1.1 Epilepsy is a common condition

People with epilepsy have epileptic seizures. These are short interruptions of the normal working of the brain. Anyone can develop epilepsy, and about one in a hundred people do. This makes epilepsy as common as diabetes or rheumatoid arthritis. Epilepsy can affect people of any age. It does not matter into which culture people are born, whether they are rich or poor, or what job they do.

Epilepsy has existed as long as mankind. It is such a common problem that there are many journals and books about epilepsy for doctors and people affected by it. There are organisations run by and for people with epilepsy, and conferences on epilepsy. Despite this, many people still do not like to talk openly about epilepsy.

1.2 There are many types of epilepsy

Seizures do not look the same in all people with epilepsy. However, one person usually has the same type of seizure all the time. Over the last 200 years certain types of seizures and epilepsy have been classified into different groups. Such categories of seizures or types of epilepsy are important because they help in the choice of treatment and they give an idea how the condition will develop over the years. Such predictions cannot be definite, of course.

Seizures are either "focal" (also called partial) or "generalised". In focal seizures, only one part of the brain does not work normally. During generalised seizures the whole brain is involved, so that normal function is interrupted in both halves of the brain. The two halves of the brain are also known as hemispheres.

The classification of seizures also distinguishes between various types of focal or generalised seizures. "Absence attacks", for instance, are seizures with brief loss of consciousness but without any unusual movements or falls. "Complex partial seizures" are attacks in which consciousness is reduced or lost, but people may perform pointless activities like licking their lips or fiddling with clothes. They can also laugh for no obvious reason.

Apart from a classification of different types of seizures, there is also a classification of different types of epilepsy. For example, Rolandic epilepsy starts in children between the ages of five and ten, often involves seizures with twitching in the face, is commoner in boys than in girls, is easily treated with drugs and settles around the time of puberty.

Epilepsy can also be classified depending on which of the four big parts of the brain (called lobes) seizures come from. For instance, it is possible to distinguish between seizures from the frontal lobes (the front part of the brain) and the temporal lobes (the parts of the brain underneath the temples). The same type of epilepsy can be classified in different ways. Rolandic epilepsy for example can also be thought of as epilepsy with focal seizures from the frontal lobes.

1.3 Seizures briefly interrupt the normal working of the brain

Seizures are short, sudden and repeated interruptions of the working of the brain. In most people they always start from the same place in the brain. Movement, seeing, and hearing for instance are processed in different parts of the brain. Thus, what happens during a seizure can show where in the brain a seizure comes from. If the seizure consists of twitching of the muscles in the face, it is likely that there is a problem in the area of the brain which deals with movements of the face. If a seizure consists of flashes of light, it is likely to take place in the area of the brain which allows us to see.

1.4 How the brain works

Like all other organs of the body, the brain consists of cells. In the brain these cells are called "neurons". They pick up information from the environment, process this information and give instructions for movement. The neurons talk to each other using fibres, which are known as axons and dendrites. The fibres carry information in the body's own language. As yet, we do not fully understand this language into which the outside world is translated in the sensory organs. Using this language, an internal picture of the world is painted within the surface layer of the brain. When we try to study this language, it seems chaotic and confusing, as if everybody is talking at the same time.

1.5 What happens in the brain during an epileptic seizure

If an area of the brain is damaged, the signals sent out by the nerve cells change. Instead of the normal apparently random chatter, the brain activity becomes even and regular. Instead of doing their own thing the single neurons fall into step with others and act together as a group. Such regular activity can cause the muscle twitches often seen in epileptic seizures. The regular activity in recordings of electrical brain activity is called "epileptic activity" or "epileptic discharges". We do not fully understand why nerve cells fall into step in this way.

During a focal seizure, epileptic activity is only found in a small part of the brain. Neurons in other parts of the brain still work normally. In a generalised seizure, cells across the whole brain fall into step for a short while. Senses, consciousness and thinking are interrupted.

1.1 Epilepsy is a common condition

Cardiac infarction concussion Chronic pain GOUT diabetes HEREDITARY DISEASEscarlet stroke Edema tuberculosis myoma paralysis Asthma fever glaucoma tumour inflammation

Anyone can get epilepsy

Anyone can develop epilepsy, and about one in a hundred people does. This makes epilepsy as common as diabetes or rheumatoid arthritis. However, people talk much less about epilepsy than about these other conditions.

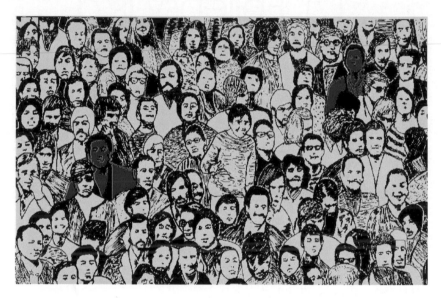

This picture shows 120 people. If they were typical of the whole population, one or two should have epilepsy. Most people with epilepsy would lead a normal life if people without epilepsy only let them. Unfortunately, many are prejudiced about epilepsy. This book is for people with epilepsy and people who live with or work with people with epilepsy. It was written to inform people about epilepsy. It is meant to explain the causes and treatment of epilepsy. It is meant to be understood by everyone.

Epilepsy is as common as diabetes or rheumatoid arthritis.

Epilepsy affects people from all walks of life

Other medical conditions, tuberculosis for instance, particularly affect poor people. There are also diseases which are more common in rich people. Epilepsy affects rich and poor alike. A person can develop epilepsy when they are a baby, a young adult or in older age.

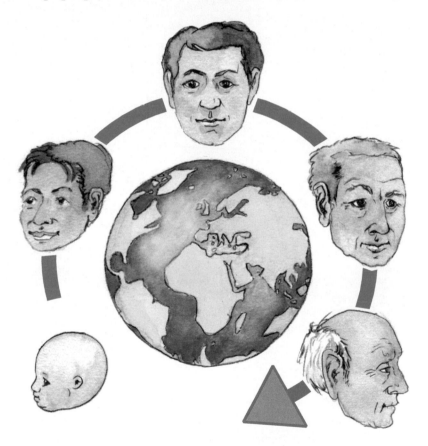

Epilepsy affects a similar number of people in all countries and cultures around the world. It has affected people for many thousands of years.

Epilepsy is described in the oldest writings

Epilepsy is as old as mankind. It is even mentioned in the first book ever written, the "Codex Hammurabi".

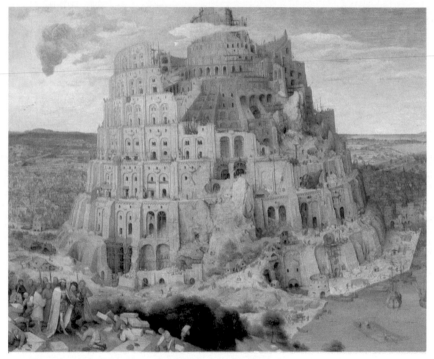

Tower of Babel, P. Bruegel the Elder, 1563 (Museum of History of Art, Vienna)

Buildings like the tower of Babel were built by slaves whose lives were not worth much and whose health was not thought of as very important. Even in those days, people knew about epilepsy. We know this from a law written down 3,500 years ago. It allowed for the return of slaves up to one month after they had been bought if they had suffered an epileptic seizure. The buyer could return a slave to his previous owner and could ask for his money back.

Epilepsy has been explained in different ways over the centuries

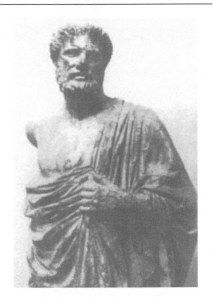

There were many theories about the cause of epileptic seizures. However, the famous Greek doctor Hippocrates knew as long as 2,500 years ago that epilepsy is no "sacred disease" but that it is caused by problems in the brain.

Many famous people had epilepsy

This includes the Greek leader and general Alexander the Great and the Russian writer Dostoyesky.

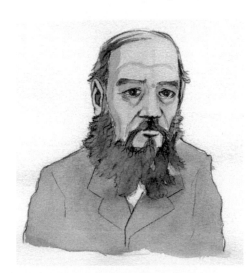

Several of Dostoyesky's books contain descriptions of people with epilepsy. When he wrote his books, Dostoyesky was using his own experiences as someone suffering from epilepsy. His seizures mostly happened at night. His wife tells us how he had a seizure at a party. After this seizure, Dostoyesky was very sad: "as if I had lost the dearest thing in my life, as if I had buried someone, this is how I felt".

There are people with epilepsy in every community

One in a hundred people has epilepsy. This means that in a village of 1,000 people, ten will have epilepsy, in a town of 100,000 people, there will be 1,000 with epilepsy.

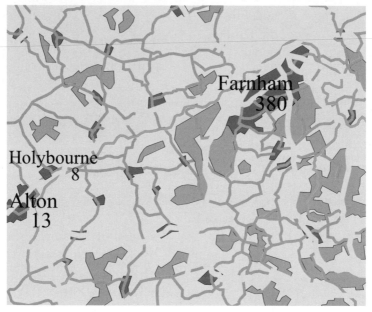

Some people join groups where they meet other people with epilepsy. Such groups (for instance the local branches of Epilepsy Action) allow people with epilepsy to learn from each other.

The numbers under each place name show how many people in these communities have epilepsy. Doctors working in these towns and villages may know about epilepsy self help groups. It is also possible to find out about groups using the addresses in the back of this book.

You can work out how many people in your community have epilepsy.

Journals about epilepsy

So many people have epilepsy that there are special journals for patients and for doctors.

The quarterly journal "Epilepsy Today" is published by Epilepsy Action. It keeps people with epilepsy in touch with each other and informs them about new medical, social, and political developments important to them.

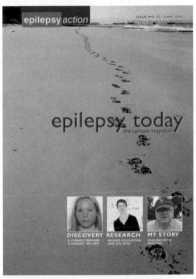

"Epigraph" is the newsletter of the International League against Epilepsy (ILAE). The League was founded in 1909 in Budapest. It has branches in many countries around the world. Apart from this newsletter, the ILAE publishes a scientific journal and organises international conferences on epilepsy. Recently, the ILAE started a campaign to bring epilepsy "Out of the shadows".

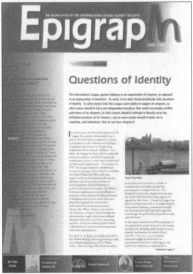

Scientific journals about epilepsy

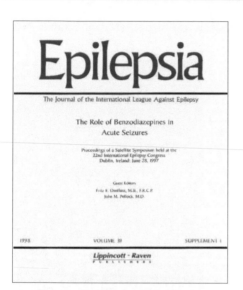

The International League Against Epilepsy publishes a journal called "Epilepsia". The picture shows the cover of a special edition of this journal telling readers about the use of "Benzodiazepine" drugs in the treatment of seizures.

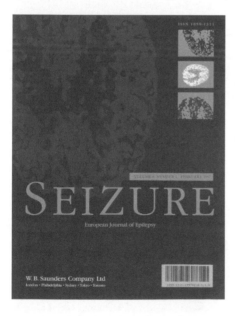

The journal "Seizure" also publishes articles which deal with epilepsy and other types of seizures. How do epileptic seizures start in the brain? How can epileptic seizures be distinguished from attacks which look like epilepsy but are not caused by epileptic activity in the brain? How should we use drugs against seizures? Such questions are also addressed in other journals like "Epilepsy Research".

Conferences for people with an interest in epilepsy

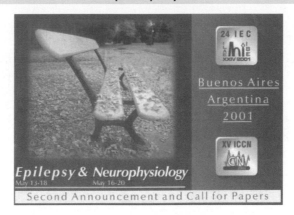

The national branches of the International League Against Epilepsy have regular meetings. The poster announces a meeting of the Argentinian Section. The main topic of this meeting was the consequences of the diagnosis of epilepsy for school-age children. There were discussions about the effect of epilepsy on performance in school and on social issues.

This poster announces an epilepsy conference in New Delhi which was jointly organised by two Asian epilepsy organisations. One of the topics discussed was "epilepsy and driving". Other issues included "women with epilepsy" and "support groups in epilepsy".

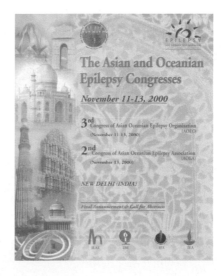

Organisations for people with an interest in epilepsy

Many of these organisations want to make the public more aware of epilepsy. They also give advice to people with epilepsy and may help them to educate their friends, family, teachers or employers about epilepsy.

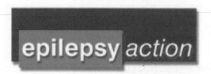

The largest epilepsy organisations in the UK are Epilepsy Action (previously known as the British Epilepsy Association) and the National Society for Epilepsy.

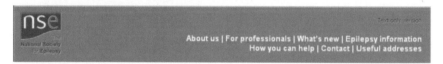

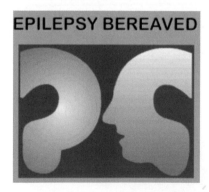

There are also organisations which concentrate on particular issues related to epilepsy. Epilepsy Bereaved for instance, helps and advises people who have lost a family member or friend because of epilepsy. This and other organisations collect money to support research into epilepsy. Addresses of organisations for people with epilepsy can be found in the back of this book.

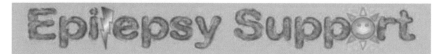

Epilepsy should be talked about more openly

Many people with epilepsy suffer more because of the wrong ideas other people have about their condition than because of their seizures.

Many countries have a special "Epilepsy Day" or "Epilepsy Week" every year to tell more people about epilepsy. The aim of such a day is to reach people who do not have epilepsy. People are addressed through television, radio, public lectures or guided tours through epilepsy centres. Everybody should know that epilepsy can affect anyone, that epilepsy is a common problem, and that people with epilepsy can work just as hard as people who do not have seizures.

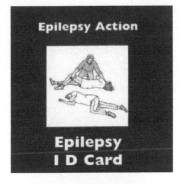

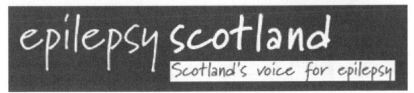

Organisations like Epilepsy Action also have volunteers who go to conferences, meetings and special events to inform people better about epilepsy.

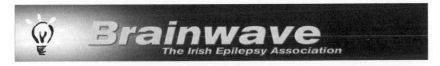

People with epilepsy have seizures. These are short interruptions of normal brain function

Epileptic seizures are not the only thing which can briefly stop the brain from working normally. Nervous twitches of an eyelid, sudden jerks whilst drifting off to sleep or shaking of the hands at times of stress are not due to epilepsy.

Sometimes it is not easy to tell whether or not an event or attack is caused by epileptic activity in the brain. Often a specialist needs to be asked for an opinion.

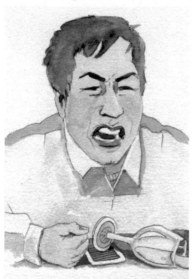
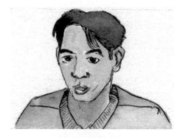
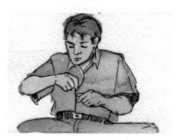

The man on the left side of the picture has an outburst of anger. The men on the right could be having an epileptic seizure. It may not be easy to tell the difference between an attack caused by emotions and attacks caused by epileptic activity in the brain.

Often interruptions of the normal brain function are not caused by epilepsy.

1.2 There are many types of epilepsy

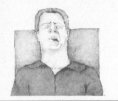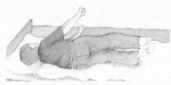

Seizures look different in everyone

Although each seizure is slightly different, seizures can be divided into different types. This is the basis of a classification of seizures which is important for choosing the best treatment.

To find out which type their seizures belong to, people with epilepsy have to answer many questions.

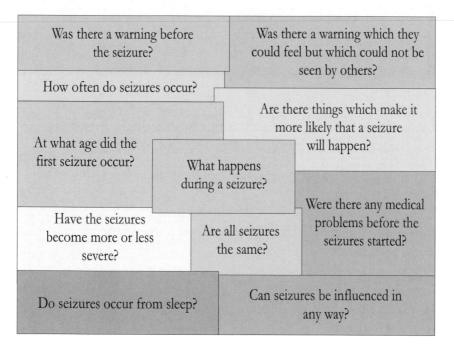

Was there a warning before the seizure?

Was there a warning which they could feel but which could not be seen by others?

How often do seizures occur?

Are there things which make it more likely that a seizure will happen?

At what age did the first seizure occur?

What happens during a seizure?

Have the seizures become more or less severe?

Are all seizures the same?

Were there any medical problems before the seizures started?

Do seizures occur from sleep?

Can seizures be influenced in any way?

Some of these questions may need to be answered by friends or relatives who have seen a seizure. What was the first thing they noticed when the seizure occurred? Do seizures end suddenly, or is recovery slow? Is there a period of confusion, tiredness or unusual behaviour after a seizure?

The answers help to identify the seizure type.

Epilepsy and seizures can be classified in a number of ways

The classification used at the moment has been developed over the last 200 years. Thanks to this classification, people who develop a particular type of epilepsy now, can benefit from the experience gained in the treatment of the same type of epilepsy in the past. If it is known for instance, that a certain drug does not work for one type of epilepsy, it makes no sense to try this drug again in someone who has just developed this type of epilepsy. Experience also helps to predict how epilepsy is likely to develop in someone over the years.

The classification of epilepsy or seizures can be likened to telling the difference between different means of transport. Although no two bicycles, cars or motorbikes look the same it is usually not difficult to separate all bicycles from all cars or motorbikes.

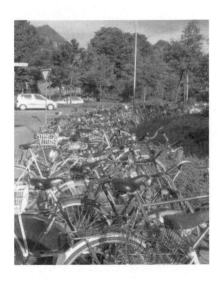

One important classification of seizures is based on changes which can be seen in the EEG. The EEG can tell whether seizures come from one particular part of the brain ("focal" seizures), or whether they involve both halves of the brain from the start ("generalised" seizures).

Seizures are either "focal" or "generalised".

In a focal seizure, epileptic activity affects just one part of the brain

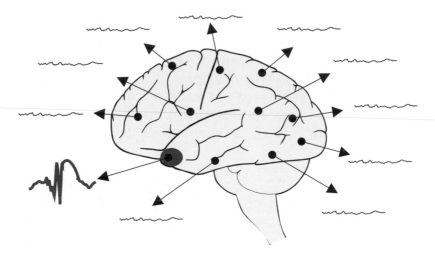

The picture shows a side-view of the brain. The wavy lines marked by arrows represent the electric activity at each of the black spots. The area of the brain marked in red is producing abnormal electric signals which are picked up by the black EEG contact. The EEG in this part of the brain shows spikes and waves. These are typical of the electric activity in an epileptic "focus". The "focus" is the place in the brain where seizures start. If epileptic activity during a seizure only affects the area around the focus, the seizure is called "focal" (or "partial"). The electric activity in all other parts of the brain is normal during such a seizure.

In principle, an epileptic focus can be anywhere in the brain. People with epilepsy may have one focus or several.

The place where seizures come from in the brain is called a "focus".

In a generalised seizure, there is epileptic activity in both halves of the brain

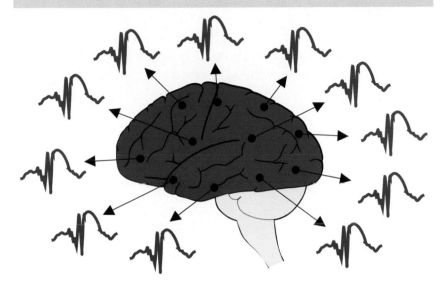

This picture shows spike and wave activity across the whole brain. If such epileptic activity is seen in all areas of the brain from the onset of a seizure, it is called "generalised". There are relatively mild generalised seizures (for instance "absence" attacks) and severe generalised seizures ("tonic-clonic" seizures). The fact that the whole brain is involved in generalised seizures does not mean that they are particularly difficult to treat. In many people generalised seizures respond to drugs more easily than focal seizures.

Any focal seizure can spread from the focus and involve the whole brain. If this happens, the seizure is called "secondary generalised". The spread of epileptic activity from a focus to the rest of the brain can take from a split second to a few minutes.

Treatment is different for focal and generalised seizures.

Tonic-clonic seizures

A tonic-clonic seizure is a major epileptic seizure. During a tonic-clonic seizure consciousness is lost and all parts of the body stiffen and jerk. A tonic-clonic seizure is frightening to see. This type of seizure has affected the way the public has thought about epilepsy for many centuries. It was often called "grand mal" in the past.

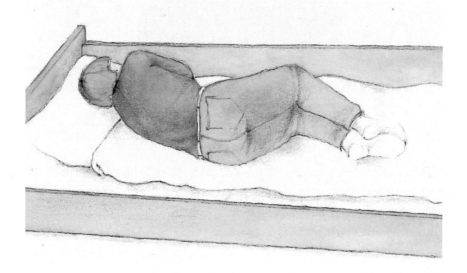

no seizure

Not everybody who has epilepsy has tonic-clonic seizures. Sometimes tonic-clonic seizures only happen during sleep. Sometimes they only happen shortly after waking up, sometimes provoked by lack of sleep. This seizure type is sometimes called "tonic-clonic seizure on awakening".

At the beginning of a tonic-clonic seizure the whole body becomes tense. As this happens, people who are standing up fall to the ground, sometimes they scream (this does not mean that these seizures hurt; people usually can not remember this afterwards). Next, the arms and legs begin to jerk in a regular fashion. The jerking first becomes more violent, then it gradually settles. During this part of the seizure, people can look blue, they can froth from the mouth, wet themselves and bite their mouth or tongue.

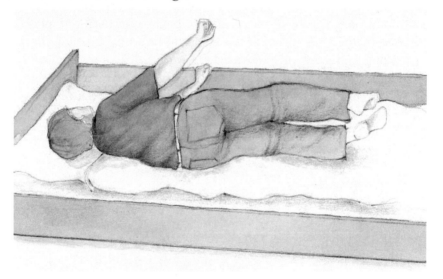

during a tonic-clonic seizure

The picture shows the first part of a tonic-clonic seizure. The body, arms and legs are stretched out (sometimes the arms and the upper half of the body are bent). The only things some people notice about tonic-clonic seizures during sleep are saliva or blood stains on the pillow in the morning, a headache or a sore mouth and tongue. They may also wake up having wet the bed or fallen out of bed.

Auras - focal seizures which cannot be seen by others

In a focal seizure, epileptic activity only affects one part of the brain. During a focal seizure which is noticed by the person having it, but cannot be seen by others, people feel, hear or see things which are not actually there, as if they have imagined them. Such sensations are called "auras". Auras can turn into other types of focal seizures which will be obvious to others if the epileptic activity spreads to an area of the brain which deals with movement or behaviour. Different people describe many types of auras. There could be a tingly feeling in one arm, seeing lights or being aware of a funny taste. An aura is felt at the very beginning of an epileptic seizure (but many people with epilepsy never have an aura which they can remember after the seizure).

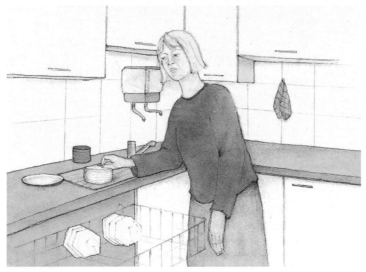

no seizure

The young woman in the picture has just come home from a busy day at work. She is loading up her dish-washer. The stress of the day is over and she is beginning to relax a little. In some people, seizures mostly occur when they are winding down.

If people have an aura before a visible seizure they can use the warning it gives them. They may go somewhere where they can be on their own if they do not want others to see their seizures, or they can sit down to stop themselves from falling over. Some people can control their brain so that an aura does not turn into a bigger seizure. They may try to think of a certain smell, bring back a pleasant memory, or rub their forearms. Usually it is a matter of trial and error to find out whether anything can stop a bigger seizure.

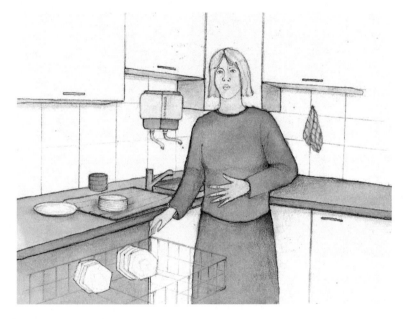

during an aura

The picture shows the young woman pressing her hand on her stomach. She has an odd sensation there and knows that she is going to have a bigger seizure. She has noticed that she can sometimes stop the seizure by concentrating on a particular song. However, this does not always work.

Tonic seizures

During a "tonic" seizure, the muscles of the body tense up for some seconds. Tonic seizures can affect the whole body or a part of the body, for instance the muscles of the shoulders and arms. Most people with tonic seizures have no sensation that an attack is coming on.

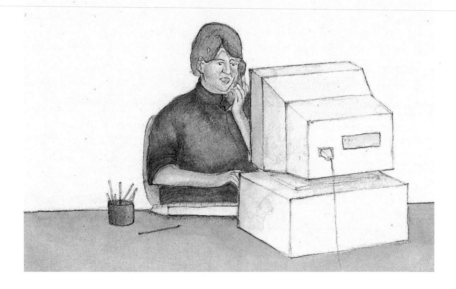

no seizure

The picture shows a woman on the telephone at work. Her tonic seizures start without warning, so that she has no time to put down the phone. The seizures always affect the arms and shoulders, they do not cause her to lose consciousness.

Tonic seizures may only affect one part of the body. For instance, they may just cause the eyes and head to turn to one side, or the stiffening of an arm and the spreading of the fingers on the same side. Consciousness may or may not be lost. If tonic seizures affect the legs, they can cause serious falls and injuries. In many people one tonic seizure is quickly followed by another. These are called serial seizures.

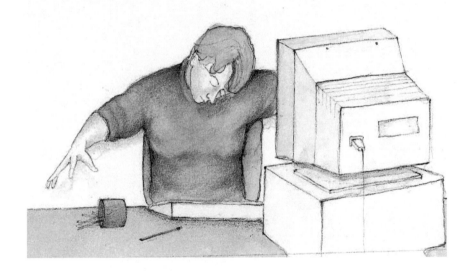

during the seizure

The woman stays in this position for a few seconds and then continues to work normally. She cannot stop the short moment of stiffening up. As her legs are not affected, her seizures do not cause her to fall.

Clonic seizures

"Clonic" means jerky. During a clonic seizure, there is regular jerking of one or several limbs. Consciousness is usually not affected. Clonic seizures usually last from seconds to minutes. Very rarely, clonic seizures cause jerking of fingers or hand lasting for years. Clonic seizures can involve any part of the body.

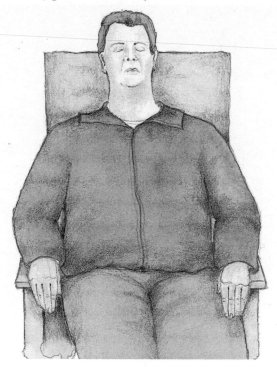

no seizure

This man had an accident several years ago. A heavy object fell on his head so that he was unconscious for several minutes. For the last two years he has had clonic seizures which he cannot stop and which often turn into tonic-clonic seizures. He is undergoing tests in the hospital to see whether the scar which the accident has left behind in his brain can be removed in an operation so that the epilepsy would stop.

One particular type of clonic seizures is called "Jacksonian" seizure. In such a seizure the jerking spreads gradually through the body, for instance from a hand to the arm and the same half of the body. This type of seizure is named after the 19th century British neurologist John Hughlings Jackson. If jerking continues for hours or days, it is called "epilepsia partialis continua".

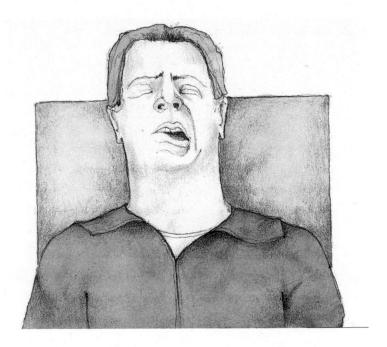

during the seizure

The picture shows a seizure during which the man has not lost consciousness. After this sort of seizure the affected body part is often weak for a while. This weakness is called a "Todd's paresis" (after the 19th century Irish physician Robert Bentley Todd).

Hypermotor seizures

During a "hypermotor" seizure, the body moves in a way which can look quite dramatic. People may scream, swear, or cry. Because of this, hypermotor seizures are sometimes thought to be "hysterical" or "psychogenic", that is a problem of the unconscious mind rather than a physical problem of the brain. Hypermotor seizures are focal seizures which start in the frontal lobes of the brain (because of this they are sometimes called frontal lobe seizure).

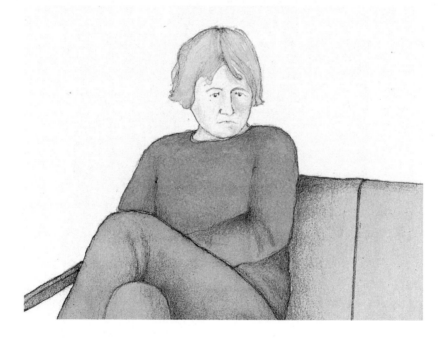

no seizure

This young woman is sitting in a waiting room. She is a little tired. Suddenly she becomes restless and the hypermotor seizure begins.

The violent movements of the hypermotor seizure affect the whole body. There may be rocking movements of the trunk, cycling movements of the legs and thrashing movements of the arms. Unlike in clonic or tonic-clonic seizures, there is usually no jerking. However, the movements of a hypermotor seizure can be so forceful that people can injure themselves.

during the seizure

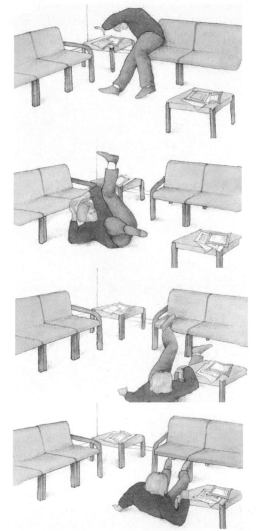

This woman is fully awake during the seizure but she cannot stop the movements although she has injured herself badly during seizures before. Hypermotor seizures often occur at night during sleep.

Complex partial seizures

In this type of focal seizure, consciousness is lost or at least reduced, and people seem to behave in an odd manner. Seizures like this are called "complex partial seizures". In the past, this sort of seizure was also known as "psychomotor seizure" or sometimes "dreamy state". Seizures like this come from the temporal lobes. People who are not epilepsy specialists often find it difficult to recognise complex partial seizures as epileptic. They may think people are just not paying attention from time to time.

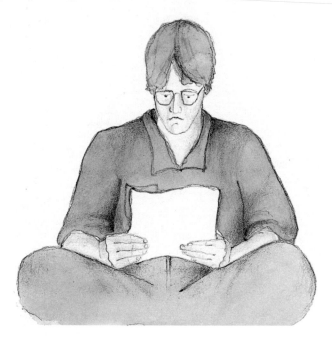

no seizure

Complex partial seizures often begin with a warning sensation (or aura). The seizure can last for some minutes and may develop into a tonic-clonic seizure. Complex partial seizures may be difficult to stop completely with drugs, so that epilepsy surgery is sometimes considered.

Complex partial seizures can involve a range of different types of behaviour. However, in each person, they tend to be the same every time. People may smack their lips, clear their throat, hum, laugh or fiddle with their clothes. Often, they seem to stare at something and cannot be distracted from it.

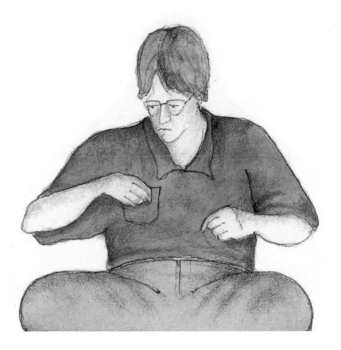

during a seizure

This young man suddenly, and for no apparent reason, has begun to play with his shirt. If he is spoken to, he will not react normally or not react at all. After one or two minutes the seizure wears off but it will take longer before he has fully recovered. He may be able to remember a warning before the seizure but not what he did or what happened around him during the seizure.

Seizures in babies

Epileptic seizures look different in babies and toddlers from older children or adults because their brain is not fully developed. There are even seizure types which are only seen in this age group. Seizures in babies are often very short.

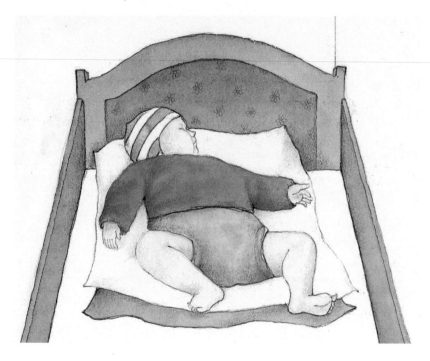

no seizure

This boy's mother noticed two months ago that he was having brief spasms of his body from time to time. Whilst he is being filmed in hospital, his blanket has been removed so that the movements can be seen better. Often there are several spasms in a row, called serial seizures. Sometimes he cries when they are over.

The best known seizures in babies are infantile spasms. They are sometimes called "jack-knife" seizures because they cause the baby to suddenly fold up like a jack-knife. These seizures are often seen in babies who have some form of brain abnormality.

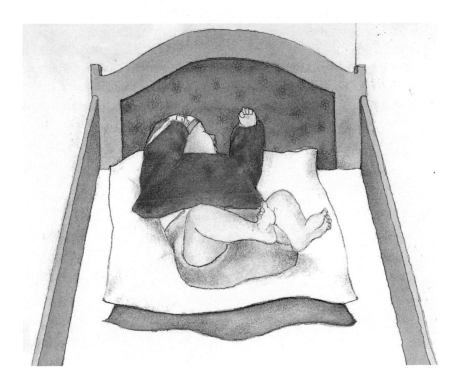

during a seizure

The photo shows a seizure during which the baby suddenly jerks, throws his arms up and bends head and chest forward. The seizure is over in seconds. Another seizure type which may be seen in babies is a tonic seizure which can last a little longer. During a tonic seizure, the arms may be raised and stretched out. Because seizures in babies can look very similar to normal movements they are sometimes difficult to spot.

Absence epilepsy of school age

"Absences" are a mild form of seizures. They consist of a short interruption of consciousness which causes people briefly to stop whatever they are doing. Absence seizures occur in "idiopathic generalised epilepsy". This is a form of epilepsy in which the whole surface of the brain produces epileptic discharges from the start of a seizure. Children who develop epilepsy between the ages of five and ten often have absence seizures. Research has shown that absence seizures are more common in girls, and that they can be treated easily with drugs. Once their absence seizures are treated, the children who have this form of epilepsy develop normally.

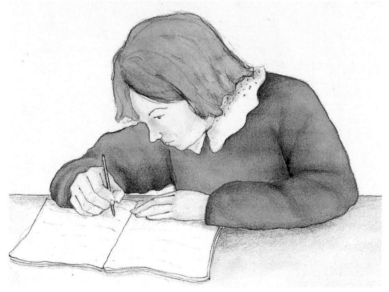

Absences may first be noticed at school. The picture shows a child trying to keep up in class.

If teachers do not know about this type of epilepsy, they often think that children are not paying attention. However, in an absence seizure children cannot react if they are told to concentrate and they have no memory for what goes on during the seizure.

Absence epilepsy often settles after a few years

Absence attacks usually disappear with low doses of drugs. After a few years the drugs can be stopped to see whether the seizures have disappeared. To do this, the dose of the drugs is reduced gradually. Drugs used for epilepsy should only be reduced with the help of a doctor as stopping medication can be dangerous without such guidance. Sometimes epileptic seizures flare up when drugs are stopped.

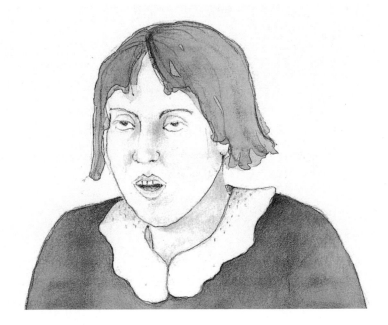

during a seizure

This girl has had a number of absence attacks in class. During such attacks she raises her head, opens her mouth, stares emptily ahead and rolls up her eyes a little. By the time the teacher tries to get her to pay attention, the attack is already over.

Absence epilepsy in teens

Absence epilepsy is a mild form of epilepsy. Seizures consist of a short loss of consciousness. Absence epilepsy in teens is one of the "idiopathic generalised" types of epilepsy. Idiopathic means that it is not clear what causes the seizure and where exactly they start in the brain. Generalised means that the whole surface of the brain produces epileptic activity during a seizure. Absence seizures tend to respond well to treatment with drugs.

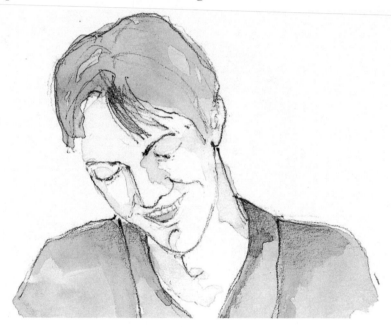

no seizure

The picture shows a young man during a conversation. There is no warning that he is going to have an absence attack. He suddenly stops talking. He does not react when he is talked to. After a few seconds, he can carry on with the conversation. People who have absence attacks are often accused of day-dreaming or of not paying attention.

During the absence seizure, the eye-lids twitch very gently. Some people roll up their eyes, turn the head or body. However, there are no violent movements or convulsions and people do not fall.

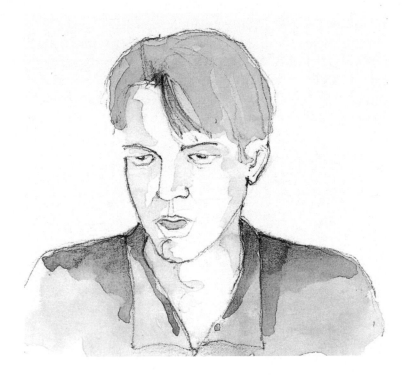

during a seizure

The picture shows the empty look during an absence attack. This young man stares ahead for about five seconds, then his eyelids twitch a little. After a few more seconds, the attack is over. He does not know that he has had a seizure although he sometimes realises that there is a brief gap in his memory, that something is missing. Absence attacks can happen very frequently in some people (many times a day) or they can be quite rare.

Rolandic epilepsy

Rolandic epilepsy makes up 10% to 20% of all epilepsies in childhood and adolescence (Luigi Rolando was an Italian 18th century physician who described the motor area of the brain where these seizures come from). Rolandic epilepsy is usually seen in children between the ages of five and ten, boys are affected more commonly than girls. Mostly, seizures can be stopped with small doses of antiepileptic drugs. Some children do not need any treatment at all. This type of epilepsy is also known as "benign partial epilepsy of childhood with centro-parietal spikes".

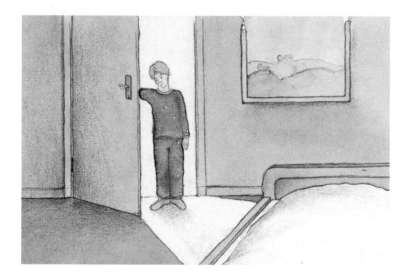

Seizures often happen in sleep. Sometimes people produce gurgling or retching noises during seizures. Saliva may flow out of the mouth. Some children are unable to speak during their seizures. Although seizures can look different in different people they are always the same in one child. Usually consciousness is not lost, although some children may seem a little slow during their attacks. Occasionally children with Rolandic epilepsy may develop tonic-clonic seizures.

Children with Rolandic epilepsy are rarely treated with antiepileptic drugs in the UK. Doctors in some other countries argue that epileptic activity could disrupt the normal functioning of the brain even if there are no obvious seizures. If this was true, antiepileptic drugs could help the brain to function better in children with Rolandic epilepsy who have few seizures but persistent EEG changes. At present, there is no clear answer to the question whether such children should be treated or not. In any event, Rolandic epilepsy usually settles at the time of puberty.

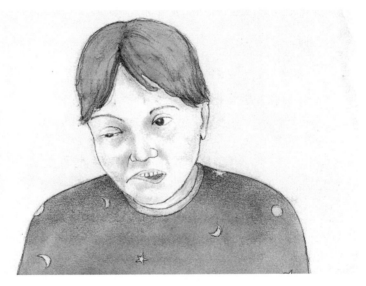

during a seizure

This child was woken up by a seizure in the early hours of the morning and has run to his parents' bedroom. He is crying because the seizure has upset him. In this child, the muscles of the right half of the face tense up during seizures.

Myoclonic epilepsy in teens

In this type of epilepsy, people have brief jerks, typically within the first one or two hours after waking up. The medical word for jerks is "myoclonus". Jerks usually affect the arms and shoulders but sometimes the whole body. People may suddenly drop a cup or their tooth brush. If the legs are affected, they may fall and injure themselves. Myoclonic seizures in teens occur most commonly together with absence and tonic-clonic seizures in "Juvenile Myoclonic Epilepsy".

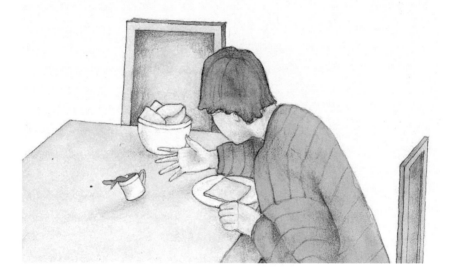

This type of epilepsy usually starts between the ages of ten and twenty. The EEG shows activity which is typical for this form of epilepsy. Often these changes can also be seen in between seizures. Apart from taking antiepileptic drugs, it is important that people with myoclonic epilepsy avoid alcohol and get enough sleep. Seizures are much more likely to happen after a late night. The risk of developing myoclonic epilepsy is in part passed down in the genes. Usually this type of epilepsy does not go away but needs to be treated for life.

Epilepsy with tonic-clonic seizures on waking up

In this type of epilepsy, people have tonic-clonic seizures shortly after waking up. Seizures only happen within the first two hours of awakening. This is so typical that most people with this form of epilepsy know that they will not have a seizure more than two hours after waking up. Sometimes they also have seizures with a short interruption of consciousness (absences) or brief jerks (myclonic seizures). Tonic-clonic seizures on waking up usually start between the ages of ten and twenty. Seizures can usually be treated easily with drugs. Most people with this type of epilepsy need to take drugs for life.

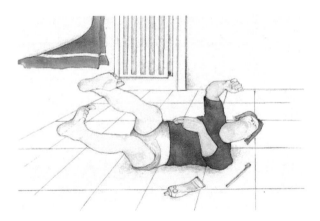

As in other types of epilepsy, little is known about the cause of seizures. It has been shown that people with tonic-clonic seizures on awakening have an unusually light sleep which can be disturbed easily. Seizures are particularly likely on a morning after a night out. If seizures in this type of epilepsy have to be observed (for instance in hospital), they are easily provoked by stopping people from sleeping. This is called "sleep deprivation". It shows that sleep is very important for people with tonic-clonic seizures on waking up. Sleeping enough and sleeping regularly can help to stop seizures.

Long seizures - status epilepticus

A condition where one seizure is followed by another is called "status epilepticus" ("epileptic state"). Any seizure can develop into status epilepticus. For instance, there is tonic-clonic status, absence status, and complex partial status. Tonic-clonic status is a medical emergency and has to be treated immediately.

A single tonic-clonic seizure

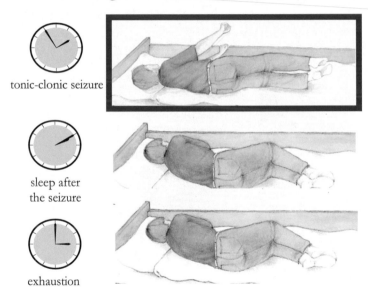

tonic-clonic seizure

sleep after the seizure

exhaustion

This picture shows a single tonic-clonic seizure which lasts about one minute. Fifteen minutes later the man is asleep. After one hour he wakes up. He feels tired and worn out, has a headache and has bitten the edge of his tongue. A single tonic-clonic seizure does not usually need emergency treatment. There may of course be exceptions to this, for instance, if someone has fallen and injured themselves during the seizure.

The picture below shows tonic-clonic status epilepticus. This is a medical emergency. Tonic-clonic seizures which go on for longer than ten minutes or which happen again after a short break have to be treated immediately, and an ambulance should be called.

Tonic-clonic status is dangerous because it stops normal breathing so that the brain does not get enough oxygen. It becomes more dangerous the longer it lasts. If tonic-clonic status lasts for over one hour, one in ten people dies, even if they are taken to an intensive care unit.

Status epilepticus

tonic-clonic seizure

second tonic-clonic seizure

third tonic-clonic seizure

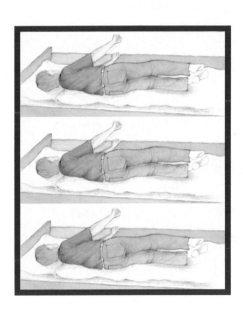

Some types of status epilepticus are difficult to recognise. People in absence or complex partial status for example may simply seem confused or slow. Such types of status are also known as "non-convulsive status epilepticus" because they do not cause tensing up or jerking of muscles. People in non-convulsive status may be able to do simple things like feed themselves or get dressed. If examined carefully, their eyelids sometimes twitch slightly. However, it often takes an EEG to find out that someone is in non-convulsive status epilepticus.

Sudden unexpected death in epilepsy (SUDEP)

"Sudden Unexpected Death" (SUD) means that someone dies suddenly (within a few minutes) and that his death is completely unexplained (no cause is found afterwards). SUD can happen to anyone. In the general population, the risk of dying suddenly and without obvious or recognizable reason is very low. The risk of dying in this way is slightly higher in babies and in people with epilepsy. When SUD occurs in babies, it is called SIDS (sudden infant death syndrome) or "cot death". When SUD occurs in people with epilepsy it is called SUDEP (sudden unexpected death in epilepsy). The risk of SUDEP increases when the following factors apply:

➡ seizures have not been stopped by antiepileptic drugs

➡ seizures over many years

➡ being male

➡ additional learning disability

➡ excessive alcohol consumption or use of illicit drugs

➡ irregular intake of antiepileptic drugs

Although SUDEP is obviously a serious event, the actual risk posed by it to a person with epilepsy is very small. People with well-treated epilepsy and good seizure control should not be worried.

It is not well understood what can be done to prevent SUDEP. A good control of seizures is helpful. This means that it is important to take antiepileptic drugs regularly and in the right doses. Too much alcohol should be avoided. When seizures cannot be stopped with drugs, epilepsy surgery should be considered.

Many questions about sudden unexpected death in epilepsy are still unanswered. Most people have died of SUDEP when they were on their own, for instance in their bed at night. However, it is likely that SUDEP is related to epileptic seizures. Several people were seen to have a seizure shortly before they died of SUDEP. The risk of SUDEP is lower after epilepsy surgery when seizures have stopped.

known causes of death	
heart disease	pneumonia
cancer	accidents
death without explanation	
SUD SUDEP SIDS	

Although epileptic seizures rarely cause people to die, the life-expectancy of people with epilepsy is a little lower than in the general population, in the same way that life-expectancy is lower with high blood sugar (diabetes). The effect of epilepsy on life-expectancy depends on how severe the epilepsy is. People with epilepsy may of course live until they are 90 or older.

Generally, epilepsy is not life-threatening.

Most people with epilepsy have seizures of one type

The classification of seizures and of epilepsy is important because it can help people to get the best treatment. If the diagnosis is childhood absence epilepsy for instance, drugs can be stopped after a few years to see whether seizures have disappeared.

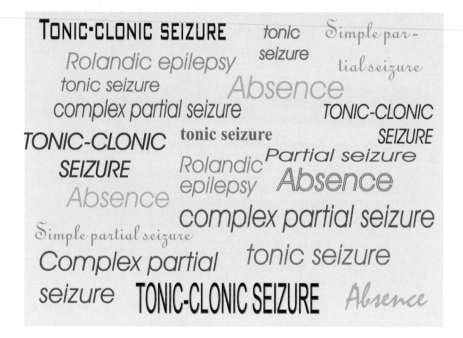

The different types of print used in this picture can be grouped together based on their colour, size or shape of the letters. In classifying seizures we first need to decide whether they are focal or generalised. Then we try to recognise the type of seizure. Finally we look whether the seizure types tell us what type of epilepsy someone has. Sometimes it is impossible to classify seizures.

In one person, all seizures tend to be similar.

1.3 Seizures briefly interrupt the normal working of the brain

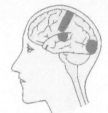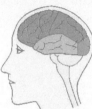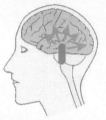

Epileptic seizures come from the brain - they interrupt normal brain function

What form a seizure takes, depends on the part of the brain it comes from. In the movement areas of the brain for instance, each area of brain deals with the movements of one particular part of the body. Brain areas are linked to the muscles by nerves. If one part of the movement area of the brain is damaged and produces epileptic discharges, jerking may be seen in the muscles that are controlled by this area of the brain.

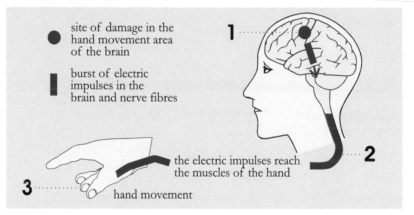

site of damage in the hand movement area of the brain

burst of electric impulses in the brain and nerve fibres

1

2

the electric impulses reach the muscles of the hand

3 hand movement

The picture gives an example. A small part of the brain (1, marked by the red dot) is damaged. Epileptic activity is produced in this damaged area. The episode (or burst) of epileptic activity runs through the nerves to the thumb (2). The thumb twitches every time a burst of electric impulses from the brain reaches the muscles in the hand (3). If the place in the brain where the impulses come from shifts a little, or if it grows and a greater area of the brain starts to send out epileptic activity, the jerking can affect other parts of the hand or the whole hand. Bursts of electric impulses are typical of epileptic activity.

The appearance of a seizure can show where it comes from in the brain.

The brain is divided into a several parts

Each half of the brain (or "hemisphere") is divided into four "lobes". They are marked in different colours in the picture.

 The frontal lobes

The frontal lobes are important for the planning and control of movements. "Hypermotor" and "Jacksonian seizures" start in the frontal lobes.

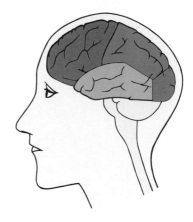

 The parietal lobes

The parietal lobes deal with sensation. Relatively few epileptic seizures start in the parietal lobes. One example are focal seizures in which people feel an odd sensation spreading over their body.

 The temporal lobes

The temporal lobes contain the "hippocampus", the "amygdala" and the hearing centres of the brain. The hippocampus is important for learning and memory, the amygdala for feelings. Both are common starting points of epileptic seizures. They can sometimes be removed in epilepsy surgery to stop epilepsy.

 The occipital lobes

The occipital lobes contain the centres of the brain which allow us to see. Seizures rarely come from this lobe. If they do, they can cause people to see flashes of lights.

All movements are controlled by the brain

Several parts of the brain are important for movements. One such area is marked green in the picture. The centres of the brain which write the programmes for complicated movements are in front of this area.

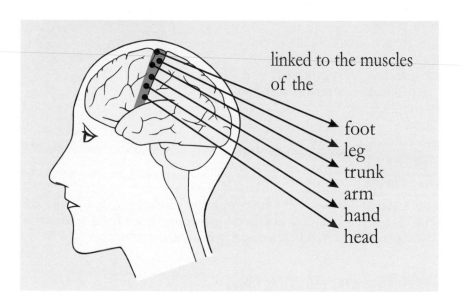

linked to the muscles of the

foot
leg
trunk
arm
hand
head

The area marked in green is linked to all muscles of the body. Parts which are close to each other within this area are linked to neighbouring muscle groups. How much space each muscle group takes up in the brain depends on how complicated its movements are. The muscles of the hand, which have to do fine and complicated tasks, and those of the face, which have to produce many different expressions, take up more space than the muscles of the thigh.

Muscles become paralysed if the centre they are linked to in the brain is damaged.

The parts of brain which directs movement can produce clonic seizures

These are seizures which consist of muscle twitching which people cannot stop. Which muscles twitch, depends on the part of the brain which is sending out the epileptic activity.

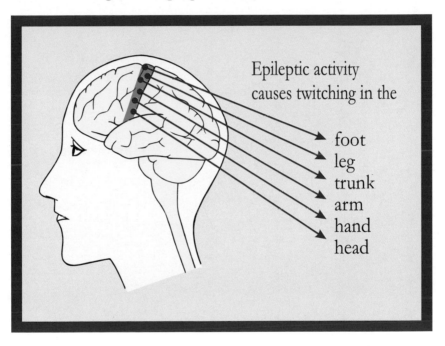

Epileptic activity causes twitching in the

foot
leg
trunk
arm
hand
head

In one person, seizures always start in the same muscles. This shows that the working of the brain is always disturbed in the same place.

When Mr K. has a seizure, his left thumb twitches about twice in one second. After a short while the twitching spreads. First, there is twitching of all fingers of the left hand, then of the whole hand. Eventually, the forearm starts to jerk, then the whole arm and shoulder. He has Jacksonian seizures in which epileptic activity spreads gradually over the surface of the brain.

Parts of the brain which are active when people feel happy, anxious or sad

The centres of the brain important for feelings are joined up in the "limbic system".

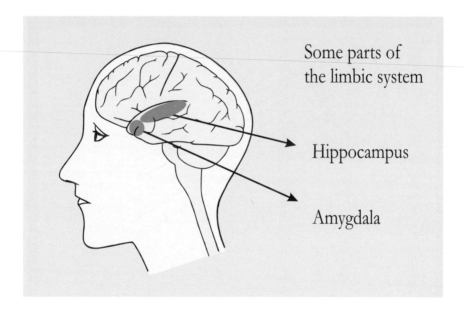

Some parts of
the limbic system

Hippocampus

Amygdala

The limbic system lies buried deep inside the brain. It is not visible on the surface. The parts of the limbic system are found in both hemispheres. This system is sometimes called the "emotional brain". It is also important for memory, however. We do not know exactly how it produces emotions like sadness, joy or anger. When it is damaged people can have emotional problems. They are more likely to become depressed or anxious than others and can find it difficult to recognise emotions in other people.

Damage to the limbic system can cause emotional and memory problems.

Focal seizures can start in the limbic system

Focal seizures from the limbic system often start with a warning (aura) of a "funny sensation" in the stomach or chest. This sensation may rise up into the throat.

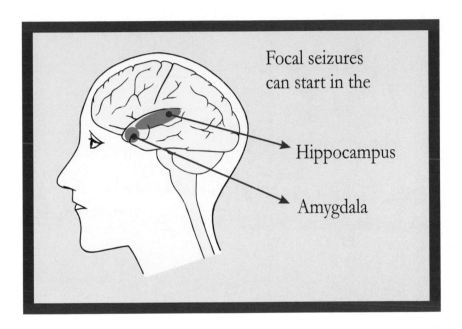

Focal seizures
can start in the

Hippocampus

Amygdala

Seizures can also start with loss of awareness. Some important parts of the limbic system are in the temporal lobes. In some people, epilepsy can be treated by removing these parts in an operation.

Mrs P. has noticed that she always has focal seizures when she feels low. She has managed to stop seizures by thinking hard of nice memories from her childhood whenever she gets the odd sensation in her stomach which she recognises as an aura.

The world outside is pictured in the brain

When the brain pictures the outside world, the information picked up by the eyes, ears and other senses is passed through the nerves to the sensation areas of the brain.

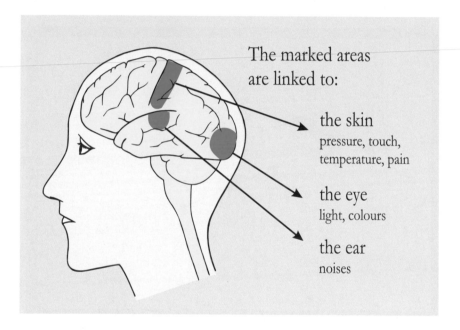

The marked areas are linked to:

the skin
pressure, touch, temperature, pain

the eye
light, colours

the ear
noises

These areas of the brain are like screens, onto which sensations from the body surface, the pictures from the eyes and sounds from the ears are projected. When you draw a letter on your skin for instance, this letter is projected onto the surface of the brain in the form of electric activity. Seeing a flash of light with your eyes causes a flash of electric activity in the vision centre of the brain. If this centre in the brain was stimulated with electric activity you would think that you had seen a flash of light, although there would not actually have been any flash. Stimulating the hearing centres of the brain would produce the sensation of hearing a noise, stimulating the skin areas of the brain a feeling of being touched.

Seizures in the areas of the brain which picture the outside world produce visions as in a dream

If epileptic activity does not spread outside the areas which deal with sensation, seizures may only consist of a perception which can, of course, only be noticed by the person having the attack.

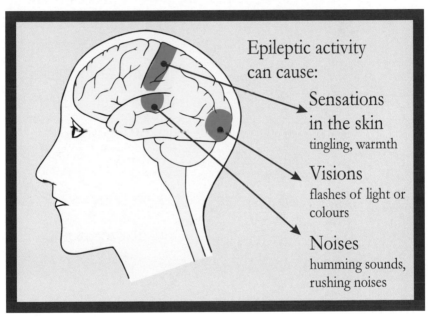

Epileptic activity can cause:

Sensations in the skin
tingling, warmth

Visions
flashes of light or colours

Noises
humming sounds, rushing noises

Epileptic seizures from these areas of the brain are called "sensory seizures". They are focal seizures which can spread and turn into tonic-clonic seizures.

Mrs L. had attacks of tingling which always affected the same spot on her right arm. She was not aware of any trigger for the tingling. Sometimes there were series of attacks. After some time, she had a tonic-clonic seizure after a series of attacks of tingling. She had a range of tests and was found to have a brain tumour. After this was removed, the attacks of tingling stopped.

The reticular formation can switch attention on or off

Hearing or seeing things does not just depend on the hearing or vision centres of the brain. The brain also has to switch these centres on. One important part of the brain which is involved in setting the level of attention paid to something or the level of concentration on something is the "reticular formation".

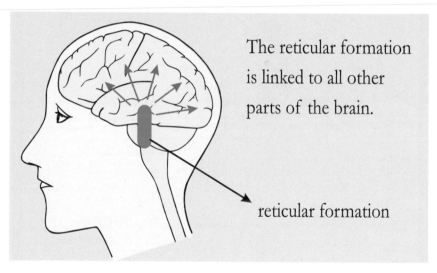

The reticular formation is linked to all other parts of the brain.

reticular formation

People can only see, hear and feel things if their reticular formation enables them to pay attention to lights, sounds or sensations. If you are watching a film and you switch your attention from the pictures to the music, you do this by switching the activity of the reticular formation from the vision to the hearing centres of the brain. The reticular formation also plays an important role in waking us up in the mornings. People whose reticular formation has been damaged are very sleepy.

Wakefulness depends on the reticular formation.

The reticular formation plays an important role in generalised seizures

Given its good connections with the other parts of the brain, it is easy to imagine how epileptic activity can spread from the reticular formation to both hemispheres. Seizures happen most readily when people are tired. In some people, seizures also start shortly after they have fallen asleep or shortly after waking up.

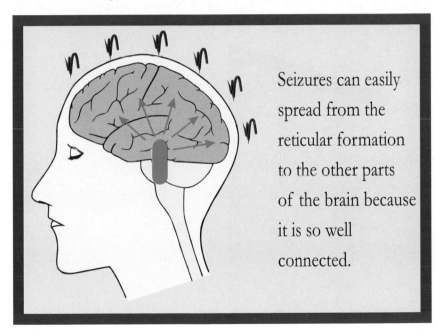

Seizures can easily spread from the reticular formation to the other parts of the brain because it is so well connected.

The picture shows how an absence seizure starts in the reticular formation during light sleep. The EEG shows epileptic spike and wave activity over the whole brain.

Mr D. has noticed that his seizures are more likely to strike when he has not slept very much or when he has had a lie-in at the weekend. He now tries to reduce the number of seizures by going to bed and getting up at the same time every day.

In many patients with epilepsy, only one small part of the brain does not work

Epileptic seizures stop the damaged area from working normally from time to time. The appearance of seizures from a damaged part of the brain is similar each time. They cause the same movements or perceptions, time and time again. We can learn a lot about how the healthy brain works from the description people with epilepsy give of their seizures or from observing epileptic seizures.

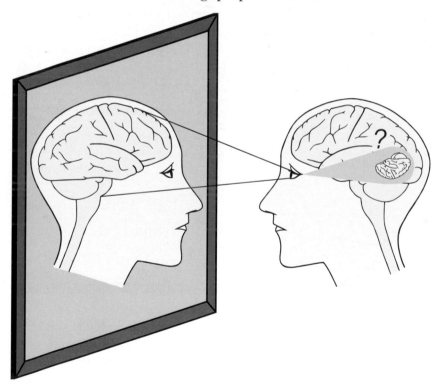

However, we still have much to learn about the working of the brain. It is fascinating to consider that in this research, one brain examines another. An organ studies itself.

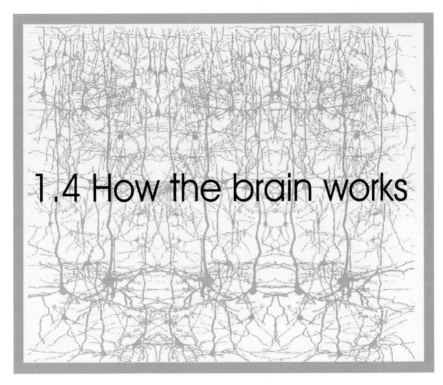

1.4 How the brain works

The brain receives signals from the body and the outside world and reacts to them

The eyes translate light signals into electric signals. These electric signals are sent to the brain through the nerves. The brain's answer mainly goes out to the muscles. For example, the head may turn towards the source of the light.

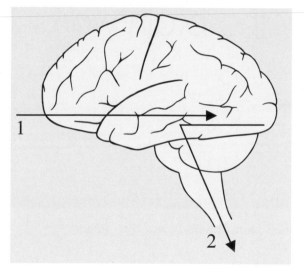

The electric impulses from the eyes tell the brain where in the outside world light and colours are. The brain uses this information to make a picture of the real world, which is similar to a photograph.

1: Signals from the outside world are sent into the brain. 2: The brain reacts to the signals from the outside world by sending commands to the muscles.

Much is known about how the eyes or ears translate light or sounds into electric signals, and how these signals travel to the brain. The brain translates millions of electric impulses back into a picture of the outside world.

During a seizure the normal electrical activity of the brain is replaced by epileptic activity.

The brain consists of 20,000,000,000 nerve cells

Many of these nerve cells are found in the surface of the brain, within an outer layer called "cortex" (this means "bark of a tree"). To see these nerve cells, microscopes have to be used.

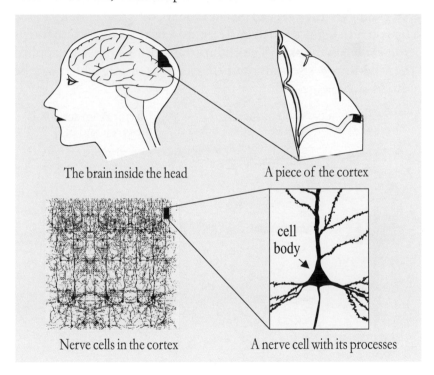

The brain inside the head

A piece of the cortex

Nerve cells in the cortex

A nerve cell with its processes

cell body

The top left part of the picture shows the position of the brain inside the head. The area marked in black is shown on the right. An enlarged slice (as it is seen through a microscope) is printed at the bottom on the left. The area marked in black is enlarged further in the bottom-row panel on the right. This panel shows a nerve cell with its body and processes (fibres). The fibres have grown out of the cell body. They pick up electric impulses from other nerve cells and pass them on.

The sensory organs translate light, sound, touch, or heat into electric tension

Nerve cells in sensory organs (like the eyes, ears and the skin) have fibres with specialised endings. Such endings pick up a signal from the outside world and translate it into a small amount of electric tension. Nerve endings in the ears can pick up sound, different endings in the eye or skin turn light or touch into electric tension. The picture shows a nerve ending in the skin. The ending transforms a pressure applied to the skin into a small amount of electric tension which can be measured as a voltage.

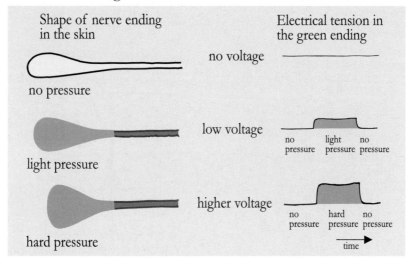

Under light pressure, the skin and the nerve endings in the skin are pulled slightly out of shape. The harder the pressure, the more the nerve endings are pulled. Changing the shape of the ending causes an electric tension, which appears in the nerve fibre marked in green. If the pressure on the skin increases, so does the electric tension. The voltage of this amount of electric tension is shown on the right side of the picture. There are other nerve endings in the skin which react to warmth, and others again which produce electric tension when the skin is injured.

Electric tension is transformed into electric impulses

Before the amount of electric tension in the nerve endings can be passed on to the brain, it has to be translated into impulses. Lower voltages are turned into fewer impulses than higher voltages. The picture shows how smaller and larger electric tension is translated into impulses. These impulses are called "action potentials".

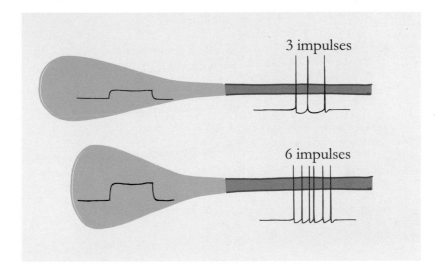

The amount of tension in the nerve endings has to be translated into action potentials because only electric impulses can travel along the nerve fibres to the brain. Impulses travel very quickly along nerves. When they arrive in the brain, they are translated back into electric tension.

The electric tension in the nerve endings can be reduced by cooling. This is why ice-spray can help to stop pain from a twisted ankle. Nerves can also be stopped from carrying electric impulses into the brain. An injection at the dentist for instance, stops you feeling pain because the pain impulses cannot reach the brain.

Neighbouring nerve endings in the skin are connected to neighbouring nerve cells in the brain

Electric impulses from two nerve endings next to each other in the skin travel next to each other in a nerve and reach areas close to each other in the outer layer of the brain. This is the "localisation principle of information processing". The picture shows how this principle works. On the left, it shows an area of skin looked at from the inside of the body.

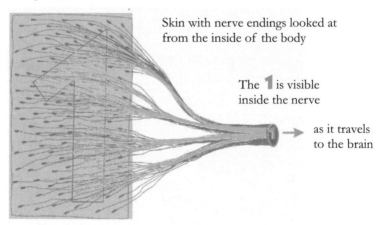

Skin with nerve endings looked at from the inside of the body

The **1** is visible inside the nerve

as it travels to the brain

The number 1 is pressed slightly onto the skin. The number is made from wood and about 10cm tall. The picture shows the area where the skin is pulled out of its usual shape by the wooden number 1. The nerve endings which build up electric tension because of the pressure in this area are marked green. The electric tension is translated into electric impulses which travel along the nerve fibres to the brain. A nerve, consisting of many fibres, has been cut through on the right side of the picture. If the fibres carrying electric impulses inside this nerve were to light up, an image of the number 1 would appear within the nerve (shown in the picture). The nerve fibres would light up as long as the wooden number 1 was pressed onto the skin.

A picture of the outside world is put together within the outer layer of the brain

Initially, the outside world (light, sound, heat, etc.) is pictured in the sensory organs. The organs produce electric tension and send it to the brain. In the brain, this electrical tension makes up a picture of the outside world.

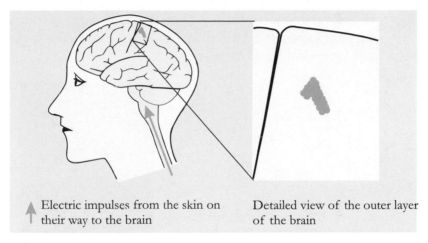

Electric impulses from the skin on their way to the brain

Detailed view of the outer layer of the brain

As an example, the wooden number 1 is pictured within the outer layer of the brain. This is possible because nerve endings from neighbouring areas of skin send their electric tension to neighbouring areas of the brain. If someone loses a leg, the area of the brain which dealt with sensations from the leg is still okay. This means that some people can still feel pain in the leg although the leg has actually gone. In contrast, when the surface of the brain linked to the leg is gone, people may feel that their leg does not belong to them, although there is nothing wrong with the leg itself. If the vision centre of the brain is damaged, people lose their vision although their eyes work normally.

Each point on the surface of the body is connected to particular points in the outer layer of the brain.

Picking up, storing and retrieving memories

The nerve cells of the brain also deal with learning and memory. It is not entirely clear how they do this. There is, however, evidence that there are two different types of memory stores, "working" or "short term" memory and "long term" memory. The working memory will only hold on to new facts for a few seconds. Everything we experience right now is contained in the working memory. Important new facts and experiences are moved to the long term memory. Having the same experience several times makes it more likely that it will be stored in the long term memory.

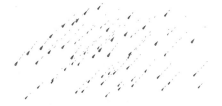

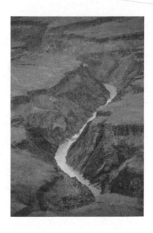

Each drop of rain leaves a small trace. Many rain drops together shape the "long term memory" of the earth.

Information held in the working memory is moved to long term memory stores by the hippocampus. It is more difficult to move information if the hippocampus is damaged in both halves of the brain. Such a problem with the storage of new memories does not change the way people experience life as it happens. They only find it harder to remember things after five minutes or two days. For instance, people who fall over and hurt themselves would normally commit the fall to their long term memory, so that they would be able to remember it later. Someone with damage to the left and right hippocampus would have just as much pain after the fall but may not remember the fall or the pain later.

Consciousness

Consciousness is the clarity with which the world appears around us. This clarity may be reduced or absent altogether. It is related to the perception of the world by the brain, not by the eyes. People can be unconscious whilst their eyes are open.

There are different types of seizures in which consciousness is reduced or lost completely. For instance, consciousness is always reduced or absent in complex partial seizures. Simple actions like laughing or fiddling with clothes may still be carried out during such a seizure, but they would not be remembered later. The pictures show how consciousness may be clouded or lost completely.

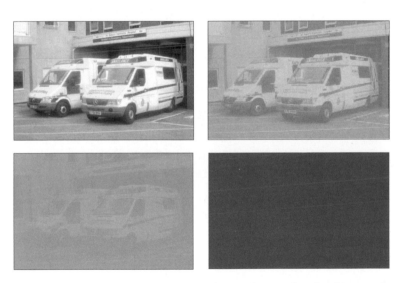

There are still many questions about how the brain produces consciousness or learning and memory. About 40 years ago it was noted that conscience could be split into a conscience of the right and left halves of the brain if the fibres connecting the two hemispheres were cut. The two halves of the brain are slightly different. In most people for instance, only the left half of the brain can produce speech, but both halves are able to read.

Normally, the nerve cells in the brain appear to chatter chaotically

There is no regular pattern of activity in the outer layers of the brain. Each nerve cell is more or less active, depending on the number of electric impulses it has received from the sensory organs or what someone is doing at the time. In the picture, electric tensions are shown as green spots. The whole surface of the brain is lit up in a shade of green. Taking a closer look, it becomes clear that different shades of green represent the outside world.

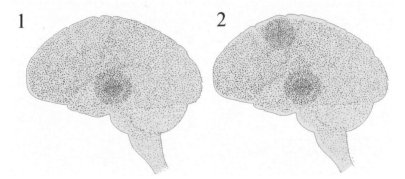

Green dots showing electric tension

The green colour is stronger in active areas of the brain. The person whose brain is shown in picture 1 is listening to music. The person whose brain is shown in picture 2 is dancing to the music, so the hearing and movement areas of the brain are particularly active.

Movements are also caused by electric tension in nerve cells, which are translated into action potentials and passed on to the muscles. The more electric impulses (or action potentials) reach the muscle, the stronger the movement.

Muscles close to each other are controlled by neighbouring areas in the brain.

1.5 What happens in the brain during an epileptic seizure?

Nerve cells normally produce electric impulses from time to time

The picture shows two series of action potentials (impulses) which come from two neighbouring nerve cells in the brain. Each upright line is one action potential.

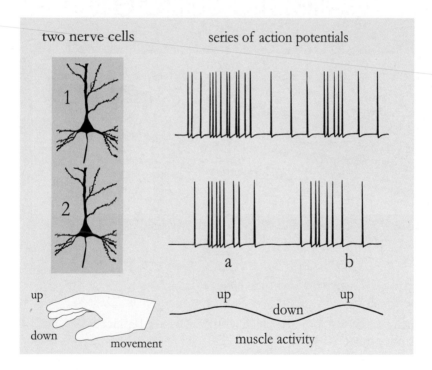

two nerve cells   series of action potentials

1

2

a   b

up   up   up

down   down

movement   muscle activity

If the nerve cells are in the movement area of the brain, the action potentials will travel to a muscle. Each action potential will make the muscle twitch slightly. Many small twitches merge into a movement. If more action potentials reach the muscle, it will tense up more strongly. The two series of action potentials can for instance travel to the muscles of a finger where they will cause the movements marked "a" and "b" in the picture.

During a seizure, normal electric impulses are replaced by epileptic activity

This picture shows two epileptic potentials of nerve cell 1 and two potentials of nerve cell 2. They are marked red. The epileptic potentials in the two cells appear at the same time.

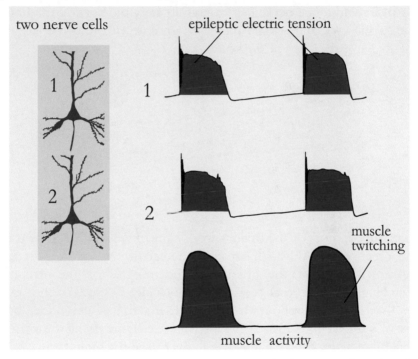

two nerve cells

epileptic electric tension

1

1

2

2

muscle twitching

muscle activity

If epileptic activity occurs in nerve cells linked to muscles, electric impulses are carried from the cells to the muscles. They make the muscle tense up (in a tonic seizure) or jerk (in a clonic seizure). Nerve cells may send out very many electric impulses to the muscles during an epileptic seizure so that muscle contraction can be very strong. Epileptic activity can affect many cells at the same time so that most muscles of the body may tense up and relax in turn. People cannot control the movements of their muscles during this sort of epileptic seizure.

During epileptic activity, all affected nerve cells are marching in step

The normal activity of nerve cells is like "chaotic chatter". In contrast, during epileptic activity, all affected nerve cells send out electric impulses at the same time and are "silent" in between.

As more and more nerve cells march in step, the area of the brain producing epileptic activity increases. In line with this, the seizure involves a greater area of the body.

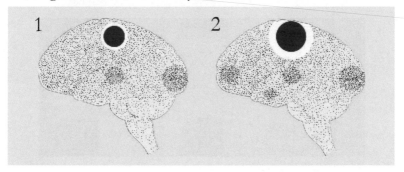

In picture 1, most of the brain is working normally. This is shown by the green dots. Although an epileptic seizure has started in the movement area of the brain, and the muscles of the arm are twitching, the person can see and hear normally. The area of the brain involved in the epileptic activity is marked in red. It is surrounded by a rim of white. This is an area in which nerve cells are trying to stop the epileptic activity from spilling over to the rest of the brain.

In picture 2, the area of the brain affected by the epileptic activity has grown. The twitching does not only affect the arm now, but also the shoulder. Over the next few seconds, the epileptic activity can shrink back. However, it can also spread further.

Epileptic activity interrupts the normal working of the brain.

Parts of the brain not affected by epileptic activity work normally during a seizure

It is possible that an epileptic seizure can cause someone to have muscle twitches or see flashes of light, but that they may have no trouble with hearing or speaking. However, epileptic activity involving only one part of the brain (as in a focal seizure) can spread to involve the whole brain. This is called "secondary generalisation".

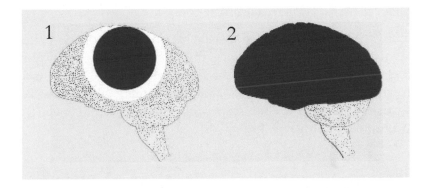

Picture 1 shows epileptic activity affecting a large part of the brain. It is marked in red. Picture 2 shows epileptic activity in both halves of the brain. If epileptic activity involves the whole brain, perception, thinking and consciousness are interrupted. There will be no memory of the seizure and no reaction to speech or touch during the event.

Most seizures stop by themselves. In some cases they do not stop and status epilepticus develops. Status epilepticus is a medical emergency. It has to be treated immediately. If a seizure goes on for longer than 5 minutes, an ambulance should be called.

It is not clear why epileptic activity starts and stops.

"Higher mental functions" of the brain and epilepsy

It is not clear how exactly the brain performs complicated tasks like perception, thinking, attention and memory, and how these tasks relate to intelligence. It is likely that many of these so-called higher mental functions of the brain are not performed by specialised, single centres in the brain, but by different brain regions working together in networks. Some people think that it will never be possible to find out how brain cells perform higher functions, because they believe these functions make up the soul.

Brain cells do not work normally when they produce epileptic activity. If epileptic activity affects the whole outer layer of the brain, all higher functions are switched off and consciousness is lost. However, when there is no epileptic activity, the brain works normally. It is therefore not surprising that people with epilepsy can do all kinds of jobs.

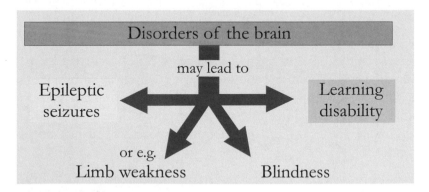

Some people with learning disabilities also have epilepsy, but epilepsy does not cause learning disability. Epileptic seizures do not damage brain cells. One exception to this is status epilepticus with tonic-clonic seizures, which is a life-threatening condition. Sometimes, however, a disorder of the brain leads to both epilepsy and learning disability.

Memory and epilepsy

Some people with epilepsy have poor memory. When epileptic seizures are caused by damage to the temporal lobes (which deals with memory functions), memory problems are more common. The temporal lobes contain the hippocampus (marked red in the picture). The hippocampus is activated when memories are moved from short term to long term stores (red lines). The hippocampus, which lies close to the centre of the skull, can be damaged when children have a high temperature and develop febrile seizures (it should be pointed out that most febrile seizures do not cause damage to the brain). The hippocampus shrinks when it is damaged (hippocampal or mesial temporal sclerosis). This makes it harder for memories to be stored.

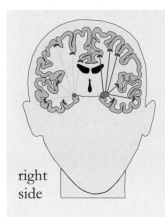

The picture on the left shows a damaged right hippocampus. It has shrunk in size and there are problems with memory.

right side

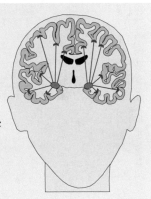

A damaged hippocampus often causes temporal lobe epilepsy. Seizures can stop when the hippocampus is removed. Operations on the hippocampus sometimes cause memory problems. Such problems cannot always be predicted before epilepsy surgery is undertaken.

Memory problems can also be caused by drugs used to treat seizures. Phenobarbital and primidone in particular are known to affect memory.

The cause of epilepsy cannot be found in everyone

At present it is only possible to identify the cause of epileptic seizures in two or three out of every ten people with epilepsy. For instance, a scar from a brain injury can cause epileptic seizures. If this is the case, epileptic activity develops around the scar. We do not know how a scar can change the way nerve cells work so that they begin to cause epileptic seizures. We also do not know why seizures from the scar only happen from time to time. Similar events in nature can help us to understand these things better.

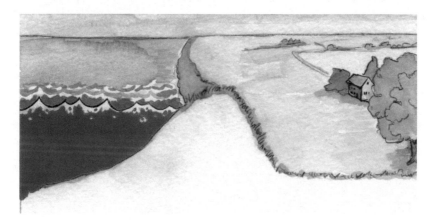

In this picture, living with epilepsy is compared to living close to the sea. Water can spill over the dam if the sea level rises, the waves become bigger or the dam becomes smaller. In this picture, the tendency to have epileptic seizures is represented by the level of the sea. If the waves are small, no water will spill onto the land (there will not be any seizures) even if the sea level is high (there is a strong tendency to have an epileptic seizure). If the size of the waves increases, a seizure may follow. You can imagine that drugs used to stop seizures have the effect of calming the waves or of building up the size of the dam.

2 Recognising epilepsy

Summary

2.1 First tests

In order to recognise epilepsy, other conditions have to be ruled out. The description of the attacks provides important clues. Even small details matter. What does the person who had the attacks remember about them? What did people see who were there at the time? If attacks happen often, people may be able to make video recordings or take photographs of them. This can be very helpful. Further clues come from the examination which may reveal pointers to a problem with the brain, or to another problem which could account for the attacks, for instance with the heart. Blood tests can help to spot conditions which cause epileptic seizures. A lack of certain vitamins, for instance, can lead to seizures which stop when the vitamins are given.

A specialist can usually work out quite easily whether attacks are caused by epilepsy or not. Sometimes, however, mistakes are made and people are diagnosed incorrectly.

2.2 EEG

The EEG is a very important test in the diagnosis of epilepsy. The recording of an EEG does not hurt and involves no risk. The EEG shows electric tension which comes from the nerve cells of the brain. The tension is picked up by small metal plates (electrodes) which are placed on the head. Each electrode shows the electric tension of the area of the brain over which it is placed. During an epileptic seizure, the electric tension in the brain has a typical pattern. The electrode which shows the typical pattern indicates that the area of brain underneath is epileptically active. However, when there is no seizure and the brain is working normally the EEG may also be normal. Thus, a normal EEG between seizures does not rule out epilepsy. Apart from being helpful in the diagnosis of epilepsy, EEG recordings can sometimes show how active epilepsy is, and how well it is treated.

The electric tension which comes from the nerve cells is very weak and can be distorted easily. Moving the eyes, chewing or using a mobile phone during an EEG, can produce so much distortion that the electric activity of the brain cannot be recognised any more.

2.3 Taking pictures of the brain

Epileptic activity often comes from a part of the brain which does not look normal. The shape or structure of the brain can be abnormal after infections, injuries, if there is a tumour, or if the brain or blood vessels have not developed well. There are several ways of taking pictures of the brain without opening the skull. "Magnetic Resonance Imaging" (MRI) takes the clearest pictures. "Computed Tomography" (CT), "Positron Emission Tomography" (PET) and "Single Photon Emission Computed Tomography" (SPECT) also produces pictures of the brain. "Angiography" is a test which shows up blood vessels.

2.4 Provoking seizures

Many people know what triggers their seizures. They may also know under which circumstances seizures normally happen. Many people may have a seizure for instance, if they have not had enough sleep. People who know what triggers their seizures can try to avoid such triggers and reduce the number of attacks.

During EEG recordings, epileptic activity is regularly provoked using flashing light (photostimulation) and overbreathing (hyperventilation). It is very unusual for one of these provocation methods to cause an actual seizure during an EEG recording but they can change the EEG pattern. This can help in the diagnosis.

Other methods of provocation may be used in hospital when people are examined to see whether they can have epilepsy surgery. If epileptic seizures are to be stopped by an operation it is important to know where in the brain seizures start. People may be kept awake or their epilepsy drugs may be stopped whilst they are wired to an EEG machine and watched by video.

2.5 Causes of epilepsy

Once it is clear that attacks are epileptic, it is important to find out what is causing the epilepsy. There are many possible causes.

Epilepsy usually develops because of a combination of two things: a lowered inborn threshold for seizures and damage to the brain. It is normally not possible to measure a person's seizure threshold but signs of brain damage can be looked for. Damage can be caused by injuries, brain tumours, infection, poor development of the brain or problems with the body's metabolism.

Damage and a low seizure threshold act together to cause epilepsy. For instance, a person with a lot of brain damage but a high threshold for epileptic seizures may not develop epilepsy, whereas someone with much less damage but a low seizure threshold does. We also know from experiments in animals that epileptic activity can be "kindled". "Kindling" may cause epilepsy in patients without any previous brain damage.

Seizure threshold changes with age. Children and older people are more likely to develop epilepsy than people of middle age.

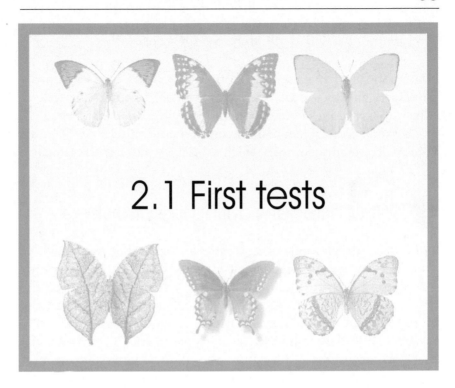

2.1 First tests

Is it epilepsy at all?

If someone first has a blackout or "funny turn" they may see a doctor for advice. The doctor will first try to work out whether the problem is likely to have come from the brain and could be a form of epilepsy, or whether it is a problem with the stomach, the muscles or the heart. There will be many questions which will help in this first assessment.

What happens during the attack?

If the attack struck suddenly and lasted no longer than a few minutes it may have been a seizure. The seizure could be caused by epilepsy or another problem. To find out the cause, a clear description of the attack is needed. What does the person remember who had the attack? Did anyone else see the attack? What did they notice? It is particular important to find out what happened from witnesses, if the attack actually caused a blackout. Were there any movements after consciousness was lost? Was the body stiff or floppy? If it was floppy during a blackout, the attack was probably not caused by epilepsy.

Are there repeated attacks?

There are epileptic seizures which only happen once in a lifetime or very rarely. An example for such occasional seizures are "febrile seizures". Febrile seizures are seizures which affect some young children when they have a high temperature. Such seizures would not normally be treated with regular antiepileptic drugs. Occasional seizures are often linked to a particular trigger, like a high temperature or lack of sleep. They are then called "provoked seizures". If the triggers are avoided, seizures may not happen at all. A diagnosis of epilepsy would only be made if seizures happened repeatedly without provocation.

Have attacks happened before?

Epileptic attacks are usually very similar in one person. If the appearance of attacks changes a lot, it is less likely that they are caused by epilepsy. Sometimes attacks are caused by stress or difficulties with handling thoughts, memories or feelings and not by epileptic discharges in the brain. Such attacks are called "non-epileptic", "psychogenic" or "functional" seizures. Some types of attack are typical for a certain age. Were there any seizures in childhood?

Does the attack spread from one part of the body?

The answer to this question can help to classify epileptic seizures into focal or "primary generalised" attacks. If the movements of a seizure start in both halves of the body at the same time, then epileptic activity usually involves both halves of the brain. This is called a "primary generalised" seizure. In a "secondary generalised seizure", the attack starts in one half of the body (and one half of the brain) but then spreads to the other.

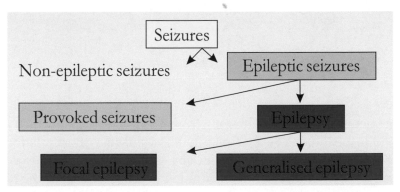

At the first visit, the doctor gets some idea of the nature of an attack. The diagram shows which decisions have to be made. Was it a seizure? Was it caused by epilepsy? Was the seizure provoked? What was the seizure type?

A good description of the seizures is very important

Every detail matters.

What happened the day before the seizure? What happened in the minutes leading up to it? Was there lack of sleep, stress or some other problem? What happened during the seizure? What did the movements look like? Were the eyes open or closed? For instance, did the seizure start with little twitches in the fingers of one hand spreading up the hand, arm and shoulder, or was there a sudden blackout without warning, followed by a fall and a convulsion? If seizures happen frequently, it is sometimes possible for friends or family members to make a video recording or to take photographs of the seizure. This can be very helpful.

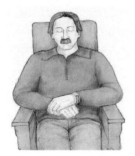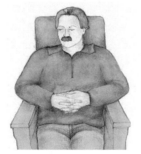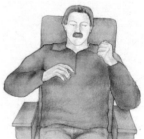

The picture shows single frames from a video recording which was made in hospital. The first picture shows a man shortly before a seizure. He is relaxing in a chair. The seizure begins in the second picture. The man has an odd sensation in his stomach. In the third picture he has lost consciousness and would not be able to answer if he was spoken to. He will also not be able to remember anything happening around him. The pictures suggest that the attack is a complex partial seizure.

Seizures cannot be stopped by an observer

An epileptic seizure cannot be stopped by people who are present at the time. Seizures will run their course and stop after some seconds or minutes. Of course, witnesses to a seizure should make sure that the person having it is safe. Things which could be dangerous, a burning candle or a piece of furniture for instance, should be moved out of the way. However, it does not help the person with epilepsy, if other people panic during a seizure. Epileptic seizures can look frightening, but it is important that people try to stay calm. If possible, observers should look at their watch and time the attack.

Absence?		
no warning	short blackout without fall	quick recovery
Complex partial seizure		
Aura, odd sensation in the stomach	not answering, fiddling, licking lips	gradual recovery
Tonic-clonic seizure		
no warning, no aura	convulsion of the whole body	exhaustion, tiredness

How people feel after a seizure depends on the seizure type. After a tonic-clonic seizure, people are very achy and tired. After a complex partial seizure, people can be confused, may not recognise their family or friends, or know where they are. This kind of confusion may not be obvious until they are spoken to. It is therefore best not to leave someone on their own after such a seizure. Absence seizures on the other hand stop as suddenly as they start. After an absence attack, people immediately know where they are, and what they were doing. A description of what happened shortly after a seizure can help to classify it.

Observation and description allow a seizure to be classified

The classification of seizures used at the moment is based on ideas developed over the last few hundred years. The diagram shows the classification of the International League Against Epilepsy (ILAE). The ILAE is an organisation of people with a special interest in epilepsy. It has branches in many countries.

Partial seizures	Generalised seizures
Simple partial seizures Motor, sensory, psychic	absence seizures (petit mal)
	myoclonic seizures
Complex partial seizures loss of consciousness	tonic seizures
	clonic seizures
Simple partial seizures with secondary generalisation	tonic-clonic-seizures
	atonic seizures
Complex partial seizures with secondary generalisation	unclassifiable seizures

The diagram shows the main headings of the classification as it was published in 1981. Today the word "partial" is often replaced by "focal" or "localisation-related". The classification helps people with epilepsy because the correct classification of their seizures makes it easier to choose a suitable antiepileptic drug. It is also important for specialists because it helps them to understand each other better when they discuss certain types of epilepsy.

A neurological examination shows whether there are other problems with the brain

During a neurological examination, the many functions of the brain (and the rest of the nervous system) are tested with very simple means. Just comparing the muscles and skin of the right half of the body with the left can sometimes give a clue to a problem with the brain. Movements may also look different on the two sides. After a stroke for instance, people may drag one leg (strokes are not caused by epilepsy, but sometimes a scar from a stroke can cause epileptic seizures). When the reflexes are tested, the tendons are stretched a little by the tap of a rubber hammer. Again, the reflexes on the right are compared to those on the left.

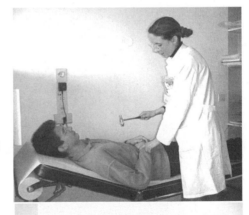

The top picture shows an examination of the reflexes. The picture at the bottom shows the finger-nose-test. In this test, the patient is asked to touch the tip of his nose with his index finger, with his eyes open at first, then with his eyes closed. In some conditions, patients struggle with this test.

Such simple tests paint a picture of the brain in the doctor's mind. Often however, the examination is completely normal in people with epilepsy.

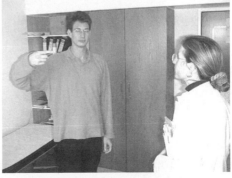

First blood tests

Blood flows through all parts of the body. When it flows through a part of the body which is not working well the composition of the blood can change. The changes can be detected and the nature of changes can provide a lead to finding the underlying disease. Several diseases including tumours, infection or problems with the body's metabolism can cause epileptic seizures. Blood tests can help to find out about such conditions.

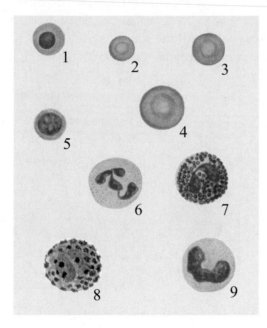

This is a picture of blood cells. Cell number one is not normally seen in the blood. The cells numbers two to four are red blood cells. These are the commonest cells in the blood. The cells numbers five to nine are white blood cells which have been stained so that one cell type can be told from another.

Some people's diet does not contain enough vitamin B. People who regularly drink too much alcohol for instance, can suffer from a lack of vitamin B. This causes the cells in the blood to change. A blood film may show red blood cells with a nucleus inside them (cell number one), red cells which are larger than usual (cell number 4) and fewer white cells than there should be. A lack of vitamin B can also cause seizures. If vitamins are given, the seizures can settle and the blood film looks normal again.

Problems with the body's metabolism can cause epileptic seizures

The body is made up of many different substances which are broken down and put together again. This constant activity (the body's metabolism) can be compared to a system of assembly lines on which more complicated substances are made out of more basic ones (picture on the left). When one particular assembly line is jammed (picture on the right), two problems arise. Firstly, there is a lack of the more complicated substance (1). Secondly, the basic substances are not used up so that they pile up in the body's tissues. If the unused material is stored in the brain, it can damage the nerve cells and cause epileptic seizures. Blood and urine tests can help to recognise such storage diseases.

Metabolism is working.　　　One assembly line is jammed.

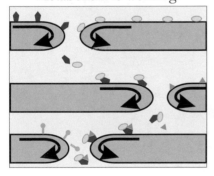 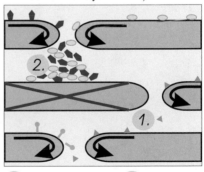

1. ◄ is missing　　2. ♪ pile up

Phenylketonuria is an example of a problem with the body's metabolism. The illness often causes epileptic seizures in the first few years of life. It affects the development of the brain. If children are put on a special diet early on, seizures can be prevented and the brain can develop more normally.

Blood tests can show whether the body's organs or metabolism are working well.

Not all seizures are epileptic

In a faint (also called syncope) there is a problem with the supply of blood and oxygen to the brain. This can cause collapses and blackouts which may look similar to epileptic seizures. However, people often feel lightheaded and queasy for several minutes before a faint, whereas there is usually only a very short warning before an epileptic seizure. People also come around much more quickly after a faint than a seizure. Sometimes a collapse and blackout can also be caused by stress or a problem with handling painful memories, thoughts or emotions. Such attacks may look quite similar to epilepsy and be wrongly treated with antiepileptic drugs for many years.

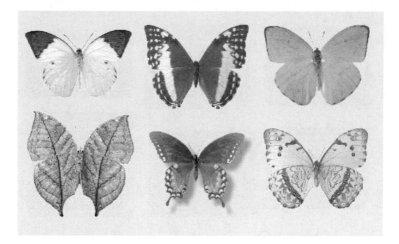

The picture shows an example of a mix up which may happen in nature. Leaves are rarely mistaken for butterflies. However, you have to take a close look not to mix-up the butterfly in the bottom left-hand corner with two leaves.

However, in most cases it is not difficult to diagnose epilepsy.

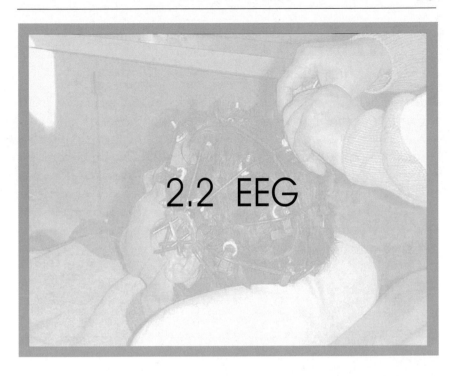

2.2 EEG

The EEG can help in the diagnosis of epilepsy

The EEG (electro-encephalogram) picks up the electric tension from the surface of the brain through small metal plates (electrodes) which are attached to the head. The EEG can be recorded on paper with a printer, or it may be stored on a computer and studied on a computer screen. A full EEG examination takes about one hour. It does not hurt and is without any risk. At first, the electrodes have to be positioned on the skin using rubber straps. A paste is rubbed into the skin under each electrode to improve the ability of the metal plates to pick up the small electric tension from the brain.

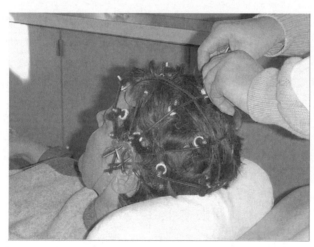

The photograph shows how a patient is prepared for an EEG recording. It is important that people having an EEG are calm and relaxed because muscle tension can hide electric activity from the brain.

What the EEG does not show:

The EEG was discovered by Hans Berger in 1932. He hoped that it would allow him to record people's thoughts. However, thoughts, feelings or intelligence cannot be measured with the EEG. When the EEG is recorded it is merely possible to see *whether* a person is thinking, not *what* they are thinking about.

Each electrode is wired to one of the ink pens of the EEG writer or one of the EEG lines on a computer. This line shows the electric tension underneath the particular electrode on the skull. If the electric tension underneath the electrode changes, it makes the line on the printer or the computer screen move so that it ends up showing a wavy line for each of the electrodes. During an epileptic seizure, the EEG shows typical epileptic activity.

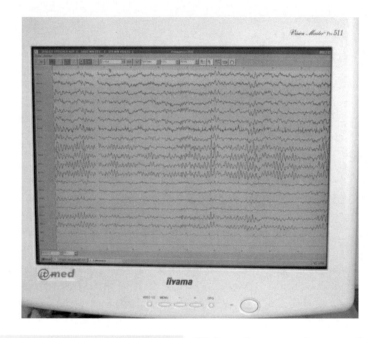

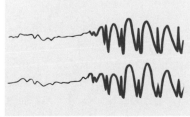

This picture shows electric tension from the brain recorded from two electrodes. The right side of the recording (the part printed in red) shows electric tension typical of epileptic activity.

The EEG is used to find the cause of attacks, to check the effect of treatment or whether changes in the EEG have settled with time.

The electric signals of many nerve cells together make up the waves of the EEG

The waves of the EEG show a typical pattern when the eyes are open and a different pattern when the eyes are closed. The shape of the waves are shown in the picture.

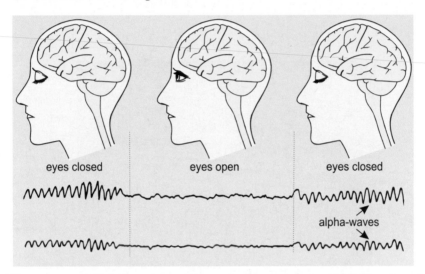

The waves, which are normally seen when someone is fully relaxed with their eyes closed, are called alpha waves. They disappear when the eyes are opened or the person thinks about something. In every EEG examination the waves are checked with the eyes open and closed.

Mr A. wanted compensation from his employer saying that he had gone completely deaf. EEG electrodes were attached to his head and a series of short noises were sent into his ears through a pair of headphones. The noises caused changes of the electric tension on the surface of the brain which were picked up through the electrodes. The fact that noises caused changes of the electric tension in the brain proved that the ears were in fact working normally.

Electric signals recorded from the head show a glimpse of the working brain

The electric tension from the surface of the brain is very weak. It can be hidden easily by other electric activity. Muscles for instance, produce much greater electric tension than the brain. When people move their eyes during an EEG recording, when they chew or swallow, the tension from the brain is hidden by the greater electric tension from the muscles. The picture shows that the EEG recorded from the scalp only picks up electric tensions from the surface of the brain.

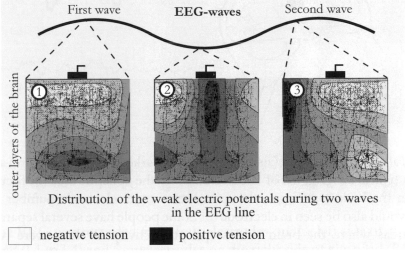

Distribution of the weak electric potentials during two waves in the EEG line

☐ negative tension   ■ positive tension

The picture shows two waves of an EEG line recorded from an electrode from one particular part of the head. The electric activity under the electrode paints an image of the outside world. If the electric tension is negative, the EEG line goes up, if it is positive, it goes down. Only a small part of the fields of electric tension with negative areas (yellow) and positive areas (blue) show up in the EEG. During the first wave for instance, the EEG only shows the negative tension on the surface of the brain (yellow) but not the positive tension underneath (blue).

Generalised epilepsy produces abnormal signals in both halves of the brain

In this picture, epileptic activity is recorded from all electrodes over the area printed red. Whilst this activity is recorded, consciousness is lost. The EEG shows a brief absence seizure. During this type of epileptic seizure, people seem to "freeze" for a few seconds.

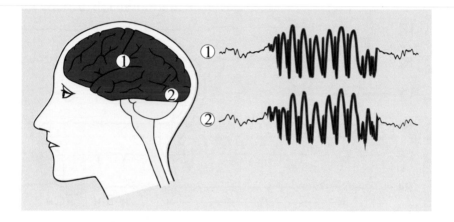

The EEG can show whether epileptic activity occurs in all electrodes from the very beginning of an attack (as in primary generalised seizures) or whether it starts in one electrode and then spreads to others (as in partial seizures with secondary generalisation). This is very important because the two types of epilepsy are treated differently.

A five-year-old girl developed short blackouts (absence attacks) during which she was unconscious but did not fall or move. During such attacks, the EEG showed the pattern of spikes and waves marked red in the picture. After she started taking antiepileptic drugs, her seizures stopped. When there had been no seizures for several years, she decided to try to reduce the medication with her doctor's help.

Twelve-year-old Paul has had brief moments for some years during which he would stare into space. He seemed to come round rapidly when he was spoken to, so his family, friends and teachers thought that he was just absentminded. Eventually Paul had a tonic-clonic seizure and underwent an EEG. This showed that his moments of absentmindedness were epileptic absence seizures.

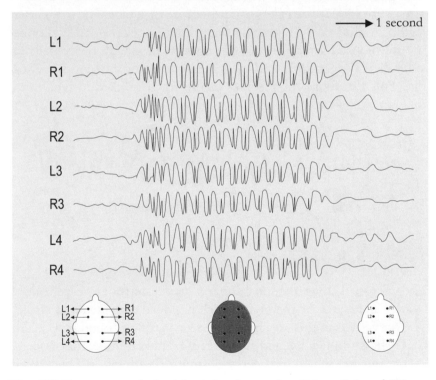

The EEG was recorded with eight electrodes (L1 to L4 and R1 to R4). The picture at the bottom of the diagram show where the electrodes were attached to the head. The EEG suddenly became abnormal in all electrodes. Paul did not answer when the technician tried to talk to him. The abnormal signals disappeared again after six seconds. Paul could not remember that the technician had tried to speak to him.

Other medical disorders can cause changes in the EEG

The EEG is mostly used to find out more about the type of epilepsy, where seizures are coming from in the brain, or how well antiepileptic drugs are working.

The EEG can also show changes in other conditions, for instance after a stroke. Most strokes occur because of a blockage in an artery leading to the brain. This means that the nerve cells normally supplied by the blocked artery do not get enough blood. If nerve cells are starved of oxygen and sugar (which are carried by the blood) they can die. This can cause the changes in the EEG marked in blue in the diagram below

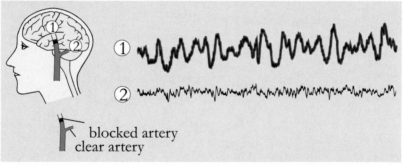

blocked artery
clear artery

The picture shows the position of two electrodes. Electrode ① "looks" at an area of the brain which has been damaged by a stroke. The nerve cells in this area have not been getting enough blood. The EEG shows typical tall and slow waves printed in blue. Electrode ② looks at an area which has been well supplied with blood. The EEG is normal.

The risk of stroke and other conditions caused by hardening of the arteries increases with age. Strokes can cause the kind of damage to the brain which may lead to epileptic seizures. Hardening of the arteries in the brain (stroke or cerebrovascular disease) are the commonest cause of epilepsy in people who first start having seizures above the age of 65.

2.3 Taking pictures of the brain

Magnetic Resonance Imaging (MRI) shows the shape and structure of the brain

"Magnetic resonance imaging" (also known as "magnetic resonance tomography") is usually called MRI. It was developed in the 1970s.

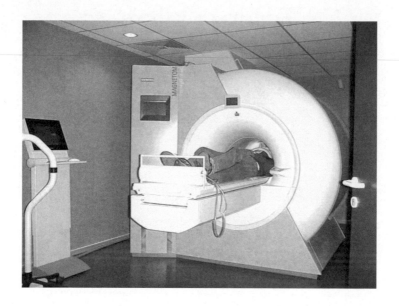

When MRI is performed, the person lies with their head inside a strong magnetic field. A scanner then measures the "magnetic resonance" of the body's tissues. A computer can turn the magnetic signals from the tissues into a picture of the skull and brain. Each picture shows a slice through the head. The head can be pictured in any direction. This means that abnormalities like scarring of the hippocampus can be seen without opening the skull, even though the hippocampus is on the inside of the temporal lobe.

Because MRI uses a very strong magnetic field, people who have a pacemaker or other magnetic metals inside their body (like some types of artificial joints or heart valves) cannot be examined with MRI. For other people, MRI is safe and painless.

MRI produces very clear pictures of the brain

MRI pictures may show small abnormalities which could not be picked up with other methods of imaging the brain. The machine takes 30 to 60 minutes to record one series of pictures. During this time, the person having the scan has to lie still in a tube which is about 70 cm wide (28 inches). Some people get anxious because there is little space in the scanner. MRI does not involve x-rays or radiation.

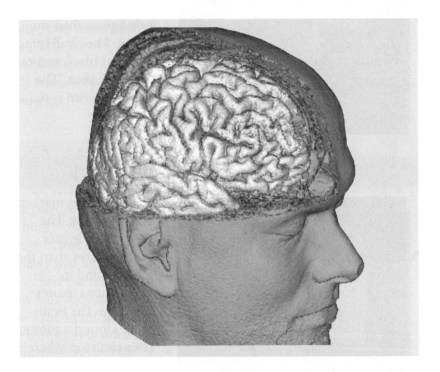

This picture of a man's brain was put together by a computer. Since the development of MRI, it has been possible to find changes in the brain in many more people with epilepsy. For example, it is now known that people with complex partial seizures often have scarring of the hippocampus in the temporal lobes.

Computed Tomography (CT) can also show abnormalities of the shape and structure of the brain

Computed tomography, or CT, uses X-rays to take pictures of the skull and brain. X-rays are sent through the head. Special cameras (detectors) pick up to what extent the rays have been weakened by the structures in the head they have passed through. The source of the X-rays and the camera travel around the head. A computer puts all measurements together and produces a picture of the head.

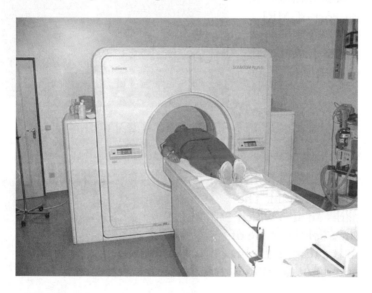

The photo shows a patient having a CT scan. The examination does not hurt and is harmless, although it does involve a small dose of radiation. A CT takes 5 to 10 minutes. It is important for people to lie still under the CT scanner because otherwise, pictures will not be clear.

CT takes pictures of the brain more quickly than MRI.

CT picture of a normal brain

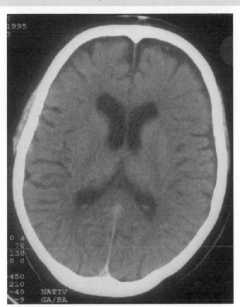

This CT picture shows a horizontal image of the brain. The skull bones show up white. The brain appears in shades of grey. The picture of the brain is less clear than that produced by MRI. In the CT harder structures look brighter than soft ones, whereas in MRI, structures are brighter if they contain more water.

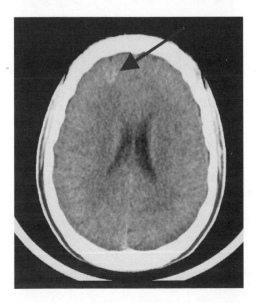

CT picture of a tumour

The picture shows a horizontal image of the brain. The arrow points at a tumour in the frontal lobe. Hypermotor seizures may start from the area of the brain around this tumour. If the tumour is removed by surgery, seizures may stop.

Occasionally, blood vessels have to be examined using angiography

When the MRI or CT pictures suggest that there may be problem with the blood vessels in the brain, these vessels can be examined by angiography. In this test, a dye, which does not let X-rays pass through, is injected into an artery. If an X-ray picture is taken as the dye is injected, the blood vessels show up very clearly.

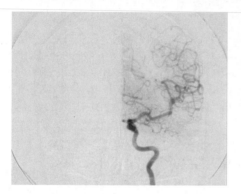

The picture shows a large artery which leads to the right side of the brain.

Angiography is sometimes used before a brain operation

An operation of the brain is possible if several conditions are met. One condition is that surgery does not damage important functions of the brain. In epilepsy surgery, speech and memory are at particular risk, because they are situated in a region of the brain in which seizures often start. The "Wada-Test" helps to show whether an operation is likely to affect speech or memory.

The test consists of two steps. At first the arteries which supply the region to be operated on are stained up with angiography. A drug is injected into the artery to put the part of the brain supplied by the artery to sleep. Then, speech and memory are tested. If the person having the test can still understand, speak and remember with a part of their brain switched off, this part can be removed without damaging these important functions.

Positron Emission Tomography (PET) is sometimes used in people with epilepsy

PET pictures show how the brain is working. To take a PET picture, a radioactive substance, for instance a type of sugar, is injected into the blood. The sugar is taken up by the brain. The radiation (or "positrons") sent out by the sugar can be picked up by a special camera outside the body. Areas of the brain which are not working well do not need much sugar, so they show up darker in this test.

The picture shows a horizontal image of the brain. The brighter the colour, the more sugar has been taken up. The outer layer of the brain, which contains the nerve cells, is particularly busy and needs most sugar. The picture shows a PET scan of a person with right temporal lobe epilepsy. Slightly less sugar was taken up by the area of the brain where seizures come from.

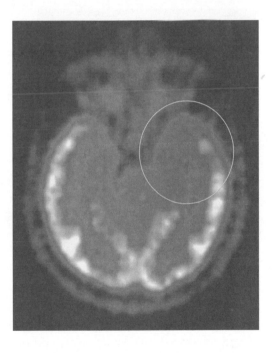

The advantage of PET lies in the fact that it shows not only the structure but also the function of the brain. The disadvantages are that the pictures are not very clear and the technique is very expensive. To a large extent, PET is a scientific and experimental method. It is occasionally combined with MRI to produce clearer pictures.

Single Photon Emissions Computed Tomography (SPECT)

To produce a SPECT picture, a substance which is radioactive for some hours is injected into the blood stream. The blood carries the radioactive substance to all parts of the body. Areas of the body which use more blood, receive more of the substance. The amount of radioactivity in the different parts of the body can be seen with a special camera.

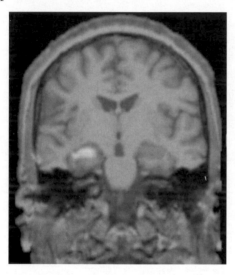

On a SPECT picture areas with more radioactivity look bright, areas with less radioactivity look dark. The total amount of radioactive material given can be very small since the special cameras are extremely sensitive.

The picture shows the result of a computer calculation in a person with seizures from the left temporal lobe. For this calculation, two SPECT pictures were taken: one between seizures and another during a seizure. Between seizures, a damaged area in the brain (like a scar) needs little blood and will show up dark on the SPECT picture. During a seizure, the area will show up bright on the SPECT picture because it uses more blood than the rest of the brain. A computer can analyse the difference between both SPECT pictures and show where any abnormalities would be found on an MRI scan. The person shown on the picture could have an operation on the left side.

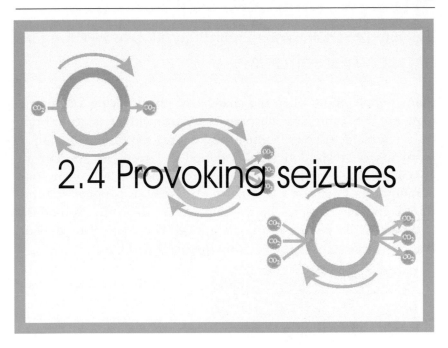

2.4 Provoking seizures

Many people with epilepsy know what can trigger their seizures

Many people know when the chances of them having a seizure is high, but they cannot usually predict seizures with certainty or bring on seizures themselves. Sometimes seizures are most common in moments of relaxation after a period of strenuous exercise or concentration, especially if people are feeling a little worn out. Sometimes a loud noise or a particular smell can trigger seizures. Rarely people have seizures whenever they do something complicated like playing a particular melody on a musical instrument. It always makes sense to try and find triggers for seizures.

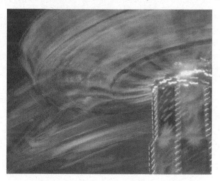

If, for instance, seizures are triggered by rapid movement, it may be best to try and avoid such movement.

People who are prone to seizures when they have not had enough sleep can try to avoid getting up very early in the morning. However, it may not be possible to avoid triggers altogether, and there is a risk that people with epilepsy avoid things which they enjoy (like meeting people or going out) although they are unlikely to bring on seizures.

Mr L. is an immigrant from Kazakstan. His family spoke English at home and he learnt to speak, read and write Russian at school. When he came to the UK he also learnt to read and write English. Now he has epileptic seizures whenever he reads an English text. He does not have seizures when he reads Russian. We cannot explain why this happens. Mr L. had to change his job because he had to read English at his workplace.

Sometimes seizures are provoked in hospital

Seizures can sometimes be brought on by "provocation" in anyone. Usually provocation is used during an EEG recording to bring out epileptic activity in the EEG. The most common methods of provocation are flashing light (photostimulation) and overbreathing (hyperventila-tion). Other methods include lack of sleep or giving a smaller dose of epilepsy drugs.

reduction of drugs   sleep
flashing lights
sleep   *Hyperventilation*
hyperventilation
s l e e p deprivation
reduction of drugs
sleep FLASHING LIGHTS

Provocation can cause epileptic seizures. However, most of the time, it only causes changes in the EEG which are typically seen in patients with epilepsy, and which suggest that someone has a tendency to have epileptic seizures. Flashing lights and hyperventilation can only provoke seizures in certain types of epilepsy. It is very easy for instance, to bring on seizures with hyperventilation in school age children with absence epilepsy.

Some people who know what triggers their seizures can avoid the trigger.

People whose seizures are provoked by flashing light have "photosensitive" epilepsy

Asking someone to look at a flashing light can help to show whether he is at risk of having photosensitive epileptic seizures. However, photo-sensitivity is only found in a small number of people with epilepsy.

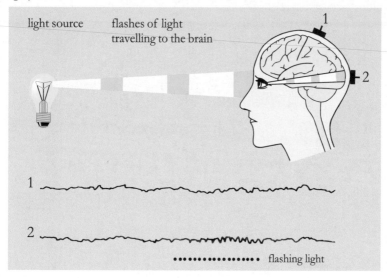

The flashes of light reach the back of the eye. They are translated into electric impulses which are passed on to the brain. Nerve cells on the surface of the brain are stimulated by each flash. In the picture, electrode ① looks at an area of the brain not involved in seeing. Electrode ② looks at the vision centre. If the brain is not prone to photosensitive epileptic seizures, the flashes will cause no or only very small changes of the EEG. In the bottom right corner of the picture, each flash is marked by a black dot. The EEG was recorded from someone who is not at risk of photosensitive seizures. The waves under electrode ② which are caused by the flashes are only small. There is no photosensitivity.

In some forms of epilepsy, flashing lights cause typical changes in the EEG

Some types of EEG changes provoked by flashing lights suggest that a person has a tendency to develop epileptic activity or is at increased risk of developing epileptic seizures.

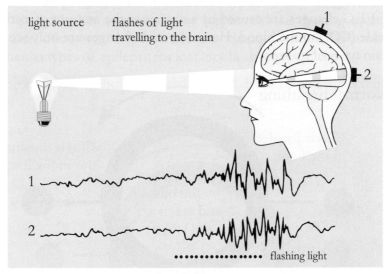

The EEG lines show waves triggered by the flashes of light. The waves get larger the longer the flashes continue. They can also be seen under electrode ①. This sort of EEG picture shows that the brain is prone to producing epileptic activity. There is increased photo-sensitivity. People who have EEG changes that are provoked by flashing lights often know that lights can bring on seizures and avoid situations where they may be at particular risk (for example in night clubs, or if they sit close to the TV). However, nine out of ten people with epilepsy are not particularly sensitive to flashing light.

In people with increased photosensitivity, the EEG can show whether treatment is working.

Hard work also causes hard breathing but does not provoke seizures

During physical work, the muscles have to work hard and use up more oxygen than when they are at rest. This means that they produce more CO_2. Breathing is increased, but only as strongly as necessary to breathe out the extra CO_2. The CO_2 level in the arteries from the lungs to the brain does not change.

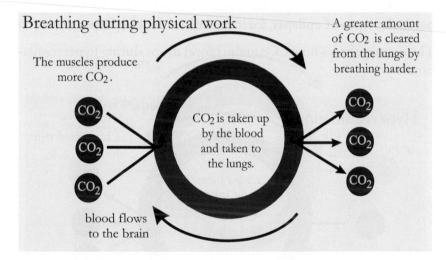

Breathing during physical work

The muscles produce more CO_2.

A greater amount of CO_2 is cleared from the lungs by breathing harder.

CO_2 is taken up by the blood and taken to the lungs.

blood flows to the brain

During physical activity, the levels of CO_2 in the arteries does not change. The risk of an epileptic seizure is not increased.

Some people begin to breathe harder than necessary when they are anxious or stressed. When this happens, the muscles and organs of the body do not produce larger amounts of CO_2 than when they are at rest. Because of the overbreathing, the level of CO_2 in the blood carried to the brain changes and the blood becomes alkaline. In some people, alkaline blood can cause epileptic seizures.

In some people, hyperventilation can cause seizures.

Lack of sleep can provoke seizures

In some people with epilepsy, lack of sleep (or "sleep deprivation") can bring on seizures. Sleep deprivation is sometimes used in hospital to find out whether seizures are caused by epilepsy, or where in the brain they are coming from. To do this, the EEG is recorded after people have been stopped from sleeping during the night.

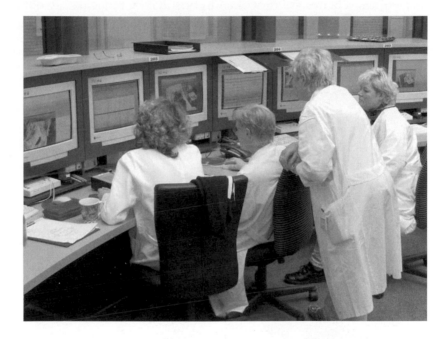

When seizures are provoked in hospital like this, patients are often not just monitored with EEG but also with a video camera. The information from the EEG and the video recording of a seizure can show where the seizure started in the brain.

The fact that seizures can be provoked by lack of sleep shows how important it is for people with epilepsy to get enough and regular sleep. Sometimes making sure that someone gets enough sleep stops seizures altogether so that there is no need for drugs.

Seizures can be provoked in several ways

During sleep, the EEG changes in a typical way. In some people with epilepsy, sleep also brings out epileptic activity in the EEG.

Seizures can be provoked by reducing antiepileptic drugs.

Sometimes seizures are provoked in hospital by reducing the doses of epilepsy drugs. This may for instance be done in people who are undergoing tests to see whether they could have epilepsy surgery.

Seizures can be provoked in many ways.

There are drugs which bring on seizures. Epileptic seizures are sometimes started with drugs or an electric current in the treatment of depression. More often, seizures occur as an unwanted side-effect of drugs. Drugs which can provoke seizures include tablets for malaria, infections, and depression. Drugs provoke seizures more easily in people with epilepsy.

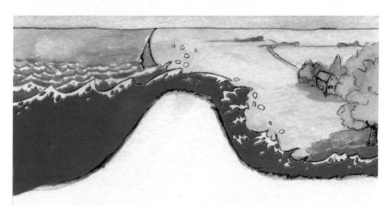

The dam in the picture may be too low, or the water too high, or the waves too large, or wind too strong. Water (as an image for a seizure) spills over onto the land. There may be one or several reasons together, why water is flooding the land.

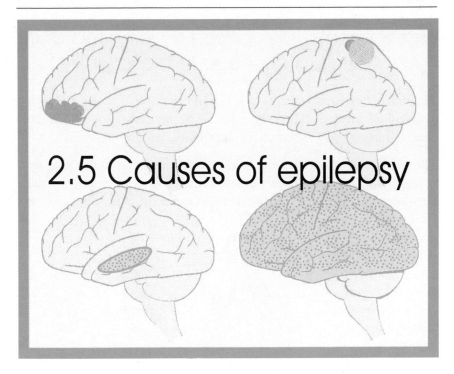

2.5 Causes of epilepsy

Epilepsy may be caused by inherited and aquired damage to the brain

The risk of seizures is different in different people. This personal risk (or seizure susceptibility) can be high, moderate or low. What determines someone's seizure susceptibility is not well known.

The EEG can provide some information about someone's seizure susceptibility when it shows many, a few or no epileptic potentials. However, the EEG cannot provide an exact measure of a person's seizure threshold.

A lower or higher seizure suscepti-bility is like any other personal trait, for instance how short, musical or hairy a person is. We do not fully understand why the personal risk of seizures varies from one person to another.

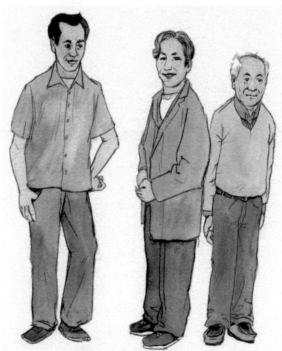

Some types of epilepsy (for instance idiopathic generalised epilepsy) are predominantly caused by inherited traits. In most people, however, a high seizure susceptibility on its own does not cause epilepsy. Epilepsy only starts when something happens to the brain. The brain can be damaged or irritated by many different causes.

Common causes of brain damage

Brain damage can, for instance, consist of a scar caused by an accident with head injury. Brain damage can also result from diseases affecting the brain.

Causes of brain damage:
- infection
- bleeding
- lack of oxygen
- brain injury in an accident
- problems with the body's metabolism
- tumour
- poor development of the brain
- interruption of the blood supply to the brain (stroke)
- abnormal aging (dementia)
- poisoning

Sometimes a combination of several types of brain damage causes epilepsy (for instance an accident and lack of oxygen).

It is not known how brain damage causes epileptic seizures.

Brain injury caused by an accident

Brain injuries can cause epileptic seizures within the first hour of having an accident, after months, or even years. More severe injuries are more likely to cause epilepsy.

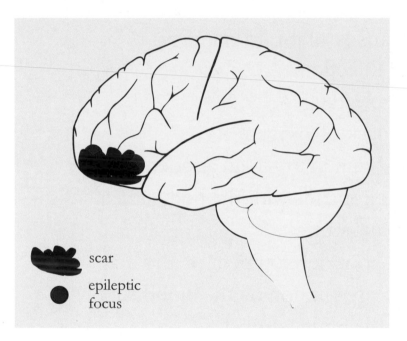

scar

epileptic focus

Brain injuries which have caused bleeding into the brain are particularly likely to cause epilepsy. However, even very severe injuries of the brain cause epilepsy in only one half of the people injured.

Mrs M. injured her brain in a car crash. She was unconscious for three days. Over the following weeks she made a full recovery. The injury has scarred over. However, one year after the accident she developed seizures which come from the brain tissue around the scar. She has to take antiepileptic drugs.

Damage caused by a tumour

A tumour presses on the brain around it. The brain cannot move out of the way because it is surrounded by the skull. This pressure may cause damage. It may also be responsible for headache and for seizures. Sometimes seizures are the only symptom of a brain tumour.

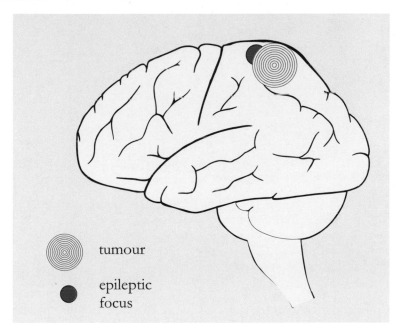

tumour

epileptic focus

It is possible that seizures will stop if the tumour can be removed by an operation.

Mr B. first had epileptic seizures five years ago which stopped when antiepileptic drugs were started. Although he continued to take his treatment, his seizures started again a few months ago. An MRI scan showed that the seizures were caused by a tumour. There is a good chance that the seizures will stop when the tumour has been removed.

Damage caused by alcohol

Stopping alcohol suddenly after drinking heavily for weeks or months can cause alcohol withdrawal. Alcohol withdrawal commonly causes seizures. However, seizures may also be caused by smaller changes in the alcohol levels in the blood (for instance when people drink more or less than they normally do).

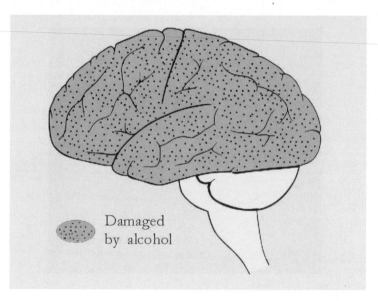

Damaged
by alcohol

Lack of sleep increases the risk of seizures further. People who have seizures because of alcohol must stop drinking if they want to get better. If people drink large amounts of alcohol for many years, the alcohol can damage brain cells so that epileptic seizures continue, even if they stop drinking alcohol.

Mr A. has had alcohol problems for 15 years. Although he has completed several alcohol withdrawal programmes, he always starts drinking again. Over the years the alcohol has damaged his brain. From time to time, this damage causes epileptic seizures. The seizures could stop if Mr A. would stop drinking.

Damage caused by "febrile seizures" - seizures related to high temperature

Fever sometimes causes seizures in babies. Occasionally, the seizures are so severe that children are taken to hospital. In over nine out of ten children, febrile seizures do not damage the brain. However, in particularly severe seizures, the combination of fever and seizures can damage the hippocampus area in the temporal lobe.

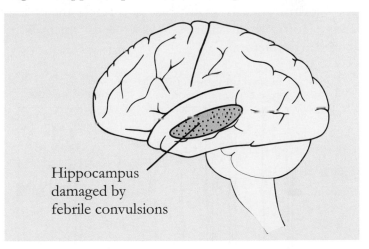

Hippocampus
damaged by
febrile convulsions

It is not known how seizures can be started by fever, how fever and seizures damage the hippocampus, and how this damage can cause epilepsy.

Mr. Z. had severe febrile seizures as a baby. Shortly after his 28th birthday he developed a different type of seizure, which could occur several times in one day. Since that time he has had frequent seizures, sometimes several in one day. The seizures always start with an odd sensation. Then Mr Z. seems to clear his throat, fiddles with his clothes and scratches around with his feet. It has not been possible to stop seizures with drugs. Three years after they first started, some seizures developed into tonic-clonic attacks. An MRI scan showed scarring of the hippocampus.

Abnormal development of the brain in the womb

During the development of the brain in the womb, some cells (printed black in the picture) act like tracks. They guide the nerve cells along the way from the place where they are made (at the bottom) to the place where they are meant to "live" and work (at the top). This means that nerve cells have to travel (or "migrate") if the brain is to develop normally. Cells which do not reach their destination sometimes form small clumps (also called "microdysgenesis", printed red in the picture).

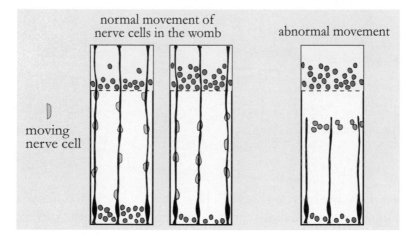

Clumps of cells which have not completed their migration are probably quite common. Only some of them cause epileptic seizures.

Mrs S. first had seizures at the age of 23. The seizures could not be stopped with drugs. She had many tests and it was thought that her seizures could be stopped by an operation. After the operation the seizures stopped but she still had to take anti-epileptic drugs. The bit of brain which was removed at surgery was examined under the microscope. This examination showed microdysgenesis.

Seizures caused by problems with the body's metabolism

The body constantly produces substances and breaks them down. All the different processes of production and breakdown together make up the body's "metabolism". Some problems with the metabolism can lead to seizures. For instance, people can develop epileptic seizures if there is not enough Vitamin B6 in the food. The seizures stop if they increase the Vitamin B6 in their food or if they take vitamin tablets. People who eat a healthy, varied diet are unlikely to develop problems because of a lack of vitamins.

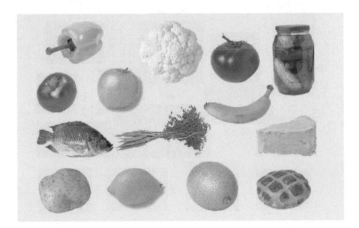

Most of us do not eat enough fruit and vegetables but eat too much fat, sugar and protein.

After birth, babies need fewer red blood cells than when they are in the womb. When red blood cells are broken down, the baby's liver produces a yellow dye. If too many red blood cells are broken down at the same time, the body may not be able to clear this dye through the bowels and the bladder. This can turn the baby's skin yellow. If the levels of the dye are very high, it can cause epileptic seizures. When the blood is cleared of the dye, the seizures stop and the skin returns to its usual colour.

Epileptic activity can be "kindled"

If the same area of the brain is irritated very slightly, for instance with a low dose of electricity, nothing happens for the first days or weeks. However, after a few weeks, an epileptic focus develops (like children who play with matches may eventually start a fire). Repeated irritation can "kindle" epileptic activity. The irritation can be electric, chemical or physical. The irritation seems to increase seizure susceptibility, that is the personal risk of seizures.

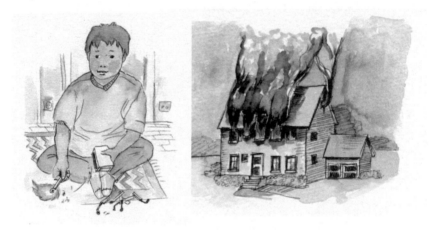

At first, a kindled epileptic focus only produces epileptic activity whenever it is irritated. However, once this irritation has caused a number of epileptic seizures, epileptic activity can also be produced when the focus is not being irritated. It seems that the focus gets stronger and stronger. Because of this, seizures should be treated as early as possible with antiepileptic drugs. Every further seizure may make it harder to stop epilepsy.

However, in many people with epilepsy, seizures do not seem to change over the years. This means that it is unlikely that the epileptic focus in these people has got any stronger.

Brain damage and inherited factors add up

In the picture, each column represents a different person. Each person has a different combination of brain damage and in-born risk of seizures (seizure susceptibility), symbolised by the two different shades of red. Where the combination of both is strong enough (that is if the column is high enough) seizures start. In person A for instance, a low personal risk of seizures and a large amount of damage add up and pass the line which shows when seizures will happen. Person C, however, has no seizures although his personal risk of seizure is much higher than that of person A.

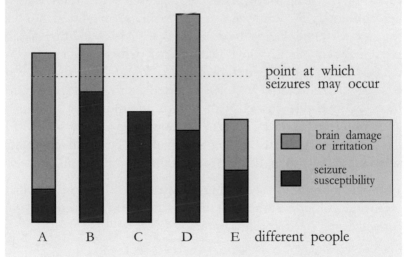

It is not understood what exactly seizure susceptibility is. It is, however, clear that an increased risk of seizures can be passed on to children from their parents. However, inherited factors often do not usually cause epilepsy on their own.

Sometimes EEG recordings of parents, brothers or sisters of people with epilepsy also show epileptic activity although they have never had an epileptic seizure. They may never develop seizures either.

The risk of seizures changes as people get older

For instance, it is higher in babies and in the elderly. A high body temperature may therefore cause a seizure in a baby but not in a young adult.

Epileptic seizures can be provoked in anyone

Everyone's brain is able to produce epileptic activity and epileptic seizures. There are certain drugs, for instance, which can start seizures. Penicillin is one of these drugs. If people take very large amounts of this drug they will develop seizures. When there were no other antibiotics 50 years ago, people with severe infections like meningitis or encephalitis were treated with such high doses of penicillin. Since only very low quantities of penicillin can pass from the blood to the brain, extremely large amounts of penicillin were used. The actual amount was just below the threshold of seizures. That is, people were treated with increasing amounts of penicillin until seizures appeared. Then the amount was slightly reduced in order not to trigger further epileptic seizures. The risk from a single seizure was smaller than the risk from meningitis or encephalitis.

Penicillin is sometimes used in animal research of epilepsy. If a drop of penicillin solution is put onto the surface of the brain an epileptic focus will develop within a few minutes.

3 Treating epilepsy

Summary

3.1 First aid during a seizure

A tonic-clonic seizure cannot be stopped once it has started. The seizure will usually stop on its own after one or two minutes. People who are present should observe the seizure and stay calm. They should make sure that the person having the seizure is safe. Dangerous objects should be removed. If the seizure happens in the street, the traffic may need to be stopped. People who continue to be unconscious after the convulsion has stopped should be turned onto their side (into the "recovery position"). If they have not fully recovered, they should not be left on their own, but should be offered help. A doctor or ambulance has to be called if a seizure lasts longer than five minutes, or if it is followed by a second seizure before the person has recovered from the first (series of seizures or "status epilepticus").

A complex partial seizure cannot be stopped either, once it has started. Since consciousness is reduced or lost, dangerous objects like knives or a burning candle should be moved away.

Febrile convulsions affect small children who have very high temperatures. High temperatures should be treated (for instance by cooling the child down or by using drugs like paracetamol) because febrile convulsions can sometimes cause epilepsy later in life.

3.2 Treatment with drugs

Antiepileptic drugs generally do not cure epilepsy, but they prevent seizures. Taking these drugs reduces the ability of the brain to produce epileptic seizures. Only in rare cases can epilepsy be cured with drugs. There are many reasons for using drugs to treat seizures. There are also circumstances when it is better not take drugs to treat seizures.

Antiepileptic drugs can stop seizures. However, we cannot say in which people a particular drug will prevent seizures. Sometimes it takes several months or even years to find the right drug, and sometimes no drug seems to work at all. One quarter of people with epilepsy have seizures which cannot be stopped with the drugs available at the moment.

Drugs enter the body through the intestines. They have to be taken up by the blood and carried to the brain. Almost all drugs are broken down in the liver. Because drugs are always broken down, they have to be replaced one or more times a day.

3.3 Antiepileptic drugs

Antiepileptic drugs are chemical substances. Most are based on substances first found in plants. There are some drugs which can work in most types of epilepsy and some which are only used in certain types. Phenytoin and carbamazepine are examples of substances which can be used for different types of seizures.

Antiepileptic drugs work on the nerve cells in the brain. They work in many different ways. Often it is not known which mechanism works in a particular person.

3.4 Side-effects

Ideally, drugs should only have the effect of stopping seizures. All other effects are side-effects. Only one patient in four ever gets side-effects. Most side-effects are only unpleasant or a nuisance. Occasionally however, side-effects are dangerous. A doctor should be asked for advice about all side-effects because it is not always obvious whether a problem is dangerous or just unpleasant. Drug information leaflets often do not explain the true size of the risk involved in taking tablets, because their main aim is to list all possible side-effects.

As drugs are carried to all parts of the body in the blood, they can have effects on all of the body's organs. Many side-effects come from the brain. Most side-effects settle on their own given time. Sometimes a drug increases the effect of another drug. One drug may also weaken the effect of another. Some antiepileptic drugs can, for instance, weaken the effect of the contraceptive pill, so that there is a higher risk of pregnancy. Alcohol can also change the effects of drugs. If people have side-effects from their medication, their treatment should be checked.

3.5 Epilepsy surgery

During operations for epilepsy, a part of the brain is removed. This means that the decision to go ahead with surgery is never made lightly. Operations are an option, if seizures cannot be stopped with drugs and if they interfere with everyday life. Before an operation, people with epilepsy have to undergo many tests. One aim of these tests is to find out where seizures start in the brain. Another important question is whether an operation would damage one of the important parts of the brain. Operations offer a chance of stopping seizures altogether.

Seizures can also be reduced by the electric stimulation of a nerve. For this treatment, an electric stimulater (similar to a pacemaker) is implanted under the skin. One of the important nerves of the body (the vagal nerve) is stimulated by this little machine through a wire. The electric stimulation rarely causes seizures to stop completely. However, the number of seizures can be reduced so that there may only be two seizures a month when there were four before. Many patients feel happier in themselves with a vagal nerve stimulator.

3.6 Other treatments which may help

Seizures are often triggered by something. If it is possible to find out what the triggers are, they can often be avoided. Sometimes this means that people have fewer seizures.

Occasionally, seizures can also be stopped by a particular activity. People often need to try out different activities to find one which can stop seizures. Some people learn to sniff a particular smell to stop a seizure from developing fully. Some people rub their forearms or think particular thoughts to stop seizures.

Obviously such methods only work if there is a warning (or "aura") before a seizure. One method which teaches people to block their seizures by controlling some of the activity in their brains is called "biofeedback".

There are also special diets which can help with seizures. The ketogenic diet has been used with particular success in children with severe epilepsy.

Acupuncture has not proven to be successful at stopping seizures.

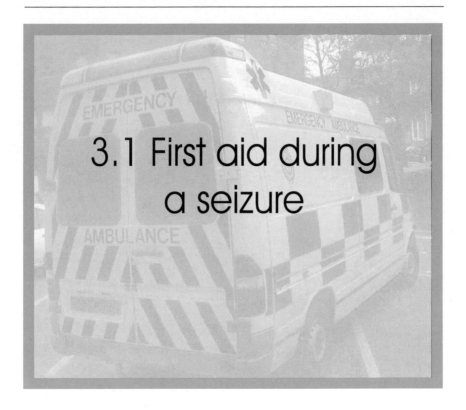

3.1 First aid during a seizure

First aid during a tonic-clonic seizure

Stay calm

A tonic-clonic seizure is frightening to see, but it is not dangerous. Trying too hard to help or panicking will only make things worse. Watching the seizure calmly and trying to notice as many details as possible (especially how long it lasts) can help with further treatment.

Do not try to stop the convulsion

The convulsion will stop by itself. Do not try to stop the movements of a seizure, or to push anything in the mouth. It does not help and can cause injuries to the person having the seizure or the person who is trying to help.

Remove dangerous objects

The person having the seizure may have to be moved away from possible dangers (like traffic, if the seizure happens in the street). Other sources of danger (like furniture, sharp objects or dangerous liquids) should be removed. Placing a cushion or some clothing under the head can stop injuries.

After the convulsion: Recovery position

If someone does not regain consciousness immediately after the seizure, it is best if they are placed in the recovery position on their side (shown in the picture below) or on their stomach. People lying on their sides or stomach are less likely to choke on saliva. Any tight clothing around the neck should be loosened to allow people to breathe more easily.

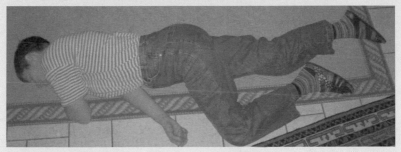

After the seizure: Stay around

Often people are quite confused when they come round from an epileptic seizure. Therefore they should not be left alone. It is better to talk calmly to them and offer help. The confusion usually settles in a few minutes.

Call an ambulance if ...

... a seizure goes on for longer than 5 minutes or if there is a second seizure without full recovery from the first. If this happens, there is a risk of "status epilepticus" and a doctor should assess the situation as quickly as possible.

You may also have to call an ambulance if the seizure has caused an injury.

Helping someone during a complex partial seizure

It is not possible to prevent a seizure from developing fully or to stop a seizure once it has started. Whilst the seizure goes on, dangerous objects (for instance a burning candle) should be placed out of reach. After the seizure, people may be confused for 10 or 20 minutes. During this time they should not be left alone. They should be watched to make sure that they do not injure themselves.

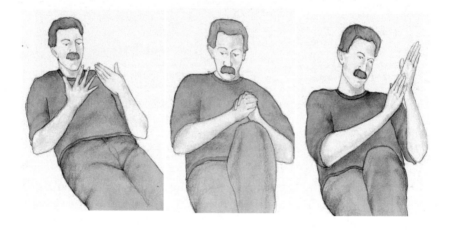

A single complex partial seizure is over after a few minutes. However, one seizure may be followed by another so quickly that the person does not "wake up" fully between attacks. This condition is called "complex partial status epilepticus" (or "non-convulsive status epilepticus"). It is not life-threatening but should be treated with drugs. Usually patients with complex partial status have to go to hospital.

Complex partial status epilepticus has to be treated by a doctor.

Seizures related to fever can be prevented by bringing down high temperatures

Babies and young children can develop a fever very quickly. Sometimes this causes "febrile seizures". Severe febrile seizures can occasionally cause epilepsy many years later. Febrile seizures are severe when they last for more than 15 minutes or happen again and again on one day. Febrile seizures are not epilepsy because they are seizures which are "provoked" by fever.

Because of the risk that febrile seizures could cause epilepsy in later life, temperatures should not be allowed to rise too highly in children under five. Parents usually learn to recognise when their child has a fever.

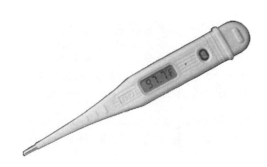

If the child shows signs of fever, the temperature should be measured. In children who have already had a febrile convulsion in the past, temperatures above 39 degrees Centigrade should be treated.

A high temperature can be brought down with drugs like paracetamol. Children can also be cooled down with cold flannels. To do this, one should soak towels in cold water and wrap them around the calves of the child. This has to be repeated every few minutes. The thermometer will show whether the temperature has gone down.

High temperatures in small children should be brought down to stop febrile seizures.

What to do to get the right kind of help?

People with epilepsy often find themselves in hospital after a seizure although they have recovered fully and feel well again. Bystanders have called an ambulance because they did not know what else to do. This would be different if people knew more about epilepsy.

- Talk to the people around you (colleagues, neighbours) about your seizures. If you do not want to use the word "epilepsy" you could always tell them about your "blackouts" or "funny turns".

- Try to explain as clearly as possible what exactly happens during your attacks and how long they go on for.

- Explain that seizures are not usually dangerous but stop by themselves.

- Tell people what you would like them to do (and what you would like them not to do) when you have a seizure.

It can be difficult to talk to people in this way. It is important to pick a good time for such a talk. However, you will find that people are much less anxious and insecure once you have told them about your attacks.

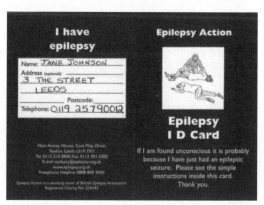

An emergency card, bracelet or locket can also help to inform people who may find you during a seizure.

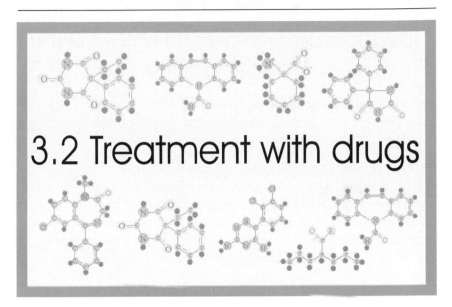

3.2 Treatment with drugs

Drugs can stop seizures, they are called antiepileptic drugs

The aim of using antiepileptic drugs is to stop seizures. This cannot always be achieved; sometimes taking antiepileptic drugs only means that there are fewer seizures.

In some people epilepsy settles completely after a while and drugs can be stopped. Often, however, antiepileptic treatment has to be taken for the long term, for years or even for life. It is important that the right dose of the drugs is taken every day. People who do not take their antiepileptic drugs regularly do not protect themselves well against seizures. Taking antiepileptic drugs on and off may even cause seizures.

Although antiepileptic drugs do not usually cure epilepsy, they protect the brain against seizures. This protection can be compared to the safety features of a car. An airbag cannot stop an accident but it can protect the driver of the car from injury.

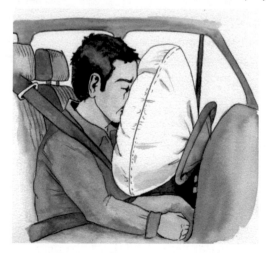

An airbag protects against injuries like antiepileptic drugs can prevent seizures. Airbags do not stop accidents, just as antiepileptic drugs usually do not cure epilepsy.

Antiepileptic drugs can stop seizures, however, they rarely stop epilepsy.

Sometimes drugs can cure epilepsy

Epilepsy can go away when seizures have been stopped for several years by antiepileptic drugs. To find out whether epilepsy has stopped, antiepileptic drugs should be tapered off very slowly, often over weeks or months. If the seizures do not come back, the epilepsy has gone. In some cases, lowering the dose of antiepileptic drugs can cause epileptic seizures to return. Sometimes it is hard to control seizures again. Antiepileptic drugs should only be tapered off under medical supervision.

Can the brain forget how to produce seizures?

We do not fully understand how people learn and how they forget. However it sometimes seems as if the brain can forget how to produce epileptic activity.

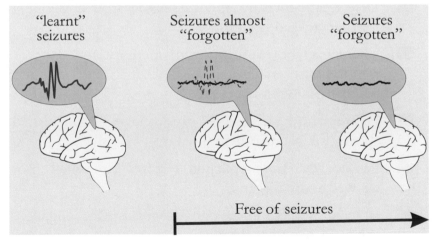

Drugs may help the brain to forget by stopping seizures. This sort of healing process occurs in some types of epilepsy but is extremely rare in others.

Any change of the dose of an antiepileptic drug should be discussed with a specialist.

Reasons for using antiepileptic drugs

Most people with epilepsy can become free of seizures if they take antiepileptic drugs. There are several reasons why it may be important for people to be free of seizures. It will depend on individual circumstances which reasons are most important. Before drugs are started it is best to talk about this with a doctor.

- Seizures can cause injuries.

- Seizures can cause problems at work, at home and they can interfere with hobbies.

- Convulsions lasting longer than 30 minutes (status epilepticus) can cause permanent brain damage.

- Drug treatment can stop focal seizures from developing into generalised seizures.

- There may be problems with memory and concentration for several hours after a seizure. This can cause problems at school or at work.

- People who have seizures cannot take part in certain sports (for instance diving).

- People who have epileptic seizures are usually not allowed to drive a car.

- If seizures occur in the bath or whilst swimming, they can cause people to drown.

- The risk of sudden unexpected death is higher when there are seizures.

- Epilepsy can sometimes be cured after it has been controlled with drugs.

Reasons against using antiepileptic drugs

People who have very mild or infrequent seizures and people with epilepsy whose seizures have not got better at all with medication may prefer not to take antiepileptic drugs. It is difficult to measure how mild or severe epilepsy is. Much depends on the circumstances of the person having the seizures.

These are examples of mild epilepsy: if there has been one tonic-clonic seizure from sleep per year for many years, or if there is twitching of the muscles of the left hand for a few minutes every week but no other seizures. A number of people would decide against taking antiepileptic drugs if they had fewer than two major seizures a year.

This is an example of severe epilepsy: if high doses of antiepileptic drugs used in combination have done little to improve seizures but are causing troublesome side-effects. In this situation some people may prefer to reduce their epilepsy treatment to a low dose of a single drug. This may cause them to have slightly more seizures but their quality of life might improve because they have fewer side-effects. A few people with severe epilepsy may even want to stop antiepileptic drugs altogether.

Further reasons against using antiepileptic drugs:

- Antiepileptic drugs can cause side-effects
- Antiepileptic drugs taken in pregnancy increase the risk of malformations in the child
- Antiepileptic drugs can change the effects of other medications

Drug treatment can be difficult and may require a lot of patience. Often the difficulties cannot be foreseen. For instance, an antiepileptic drug may not be effective even though it worked well in other people with a similar type of epilepsy. Such problems should not lead people to give up on drug treatment altogether.

Many drugs are effective against epileptic seizures

The active ingredient in a drug can stop seizures

The name of the active ingredient (also called "generic name") is printed on the box of tablets. Sometimes drugs also have a "brand name". Brand names are made up by the pharmaceutical companies which produce the tablets. Sometimes the same active ingredient is sold under different brand names. For instance Tegretol and Timonil both contain the active ingredient carbamazepine.

Tablets do not just contain the active ingredient

Pharmaceutical companies often use secret chemical processes to make the tablets they sell. They may, for instance, add substances which cause the active ingredient to be released in the small bowel rather than the stomach. This may make each tablet work longer.

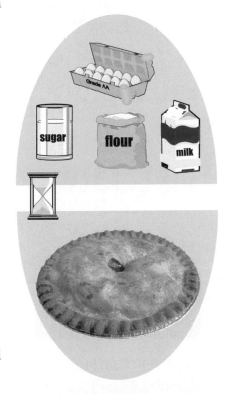

Because of such differences, tablets containing the same active ingredient can have different effects if they are made by different companies. This means that there may be problems switching over, for example, from one type of carbamazepine to another. Because of this, a drug which is working should only be changed in an emergency or after careful consideration.

Treatment with drugs may be difficult and does not always work

Research has shown which drugs work for epilepsy. However, it is never clear which drug will work in a particular person. About one half of people with epilepsy become free of seizures with the first drug they try.

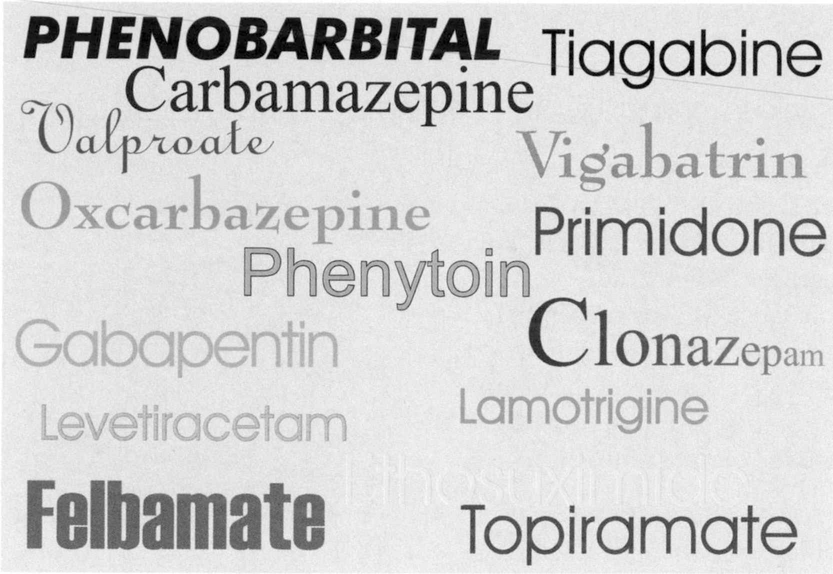

PHENOBARBITAL Tiagabine
Carbamazepine
Valproate Vigabatrin
Oxcarbazepine Primidone
Phenytoin
Gabapentin Clonazepam
Levetiracetam Lamotrigine
Ethosuximide
Felbamate Topiramate

As a rule of thumb, drugs work better if their levels in the body are higher. On the other hand, larger doses cause more side-effects. Because of this, people should use the lowest antiepileptic drug dose which stops their seizures. It can sometimes take months or years to find the right drug and the right dose. It is important that doctors and people with epilepsy remain patient in their search for the best treatment.

It is never certain whether the drug of first choice will have any useful effect.

The right drug has to be found - sometimes several drugs have to be tried

When treatment is first started for epilepsy, it is never certain that the drug chosen will actually work. However, most patients become free of seizures with the first type of treatment. If seizures continue, the dose is increased. If a drug causes unpleasant side-effects or if it does not have enough of an effect on seizures, a different drug is tried. Usually, it takes some time to switch from one drug to another.

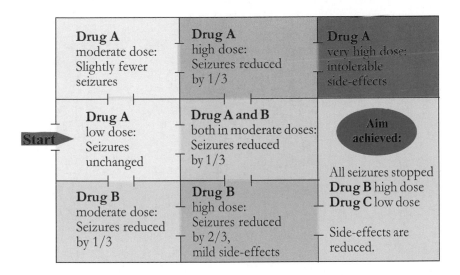

For a doctor, starting epilepsy treatment is like entering a house he has not been in before. He wants to stop all seizures. He may reach his aim immediately after stepping into the house. He may have to make his way through several rooms to the back of the house, or he may not achieve his aim at all. The example shows a type of epilepsy which usually gets better with drug A or B.

Antiepileptic drugs have to get into the brain

Once a tablet has been swallowed, it travels through the stomach into the bowels. This is where most tablets are dissolved and where the active ingredients are set free. These ingredients are taken up by the blood in the wall of the bowels and carried to the whole body in the bloodstream. In this way drugs also reach the brain where they can stop seizures.

Drugs may not get into the brain when people are sick or when they have diarrhoea. If tablets are vomited up or if the walls of the bowels cannot take up the drug, there is a higher risk of seizures.

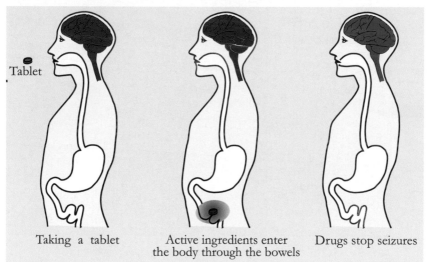

Tablet

Taking a tablet   Active ingredients enter   Drugs stop seizures
                            the body through the bowels

The strength of treatment does not depend on the number of tablets but on the dose of the drug and the amount of the drug which has entered the body. A single tablet containing 500 mg of a drug is stronger than three tablets containing 100 mg.

The amount (or concentration) of a drug in the body can be measured with blood tests.

Most drugs are broken down by the liver

The picture shows how the heart pumps blood into the brain and into the walls of the bowels. A tablet is dissolving in the bowels. The blood in the picture flows from the right to the left, past the tablet. It takes up the active ingredient (shown by the blue colour of the blood). Some of the drug never reaches the brain: it is carried through the liver and broken down there. The rest is carried past the liver to the heart. From there, it is pumped to the brain where it can stop seizures.

The drug concentration in the blood changes.

The amount of a drug in the blood is greatest in the bowels where the tablets have dissolved. The amount is smaller in the blood which arrives from the bowels in the heart because some of the drug has been broken down and passed out of the body by the liver.

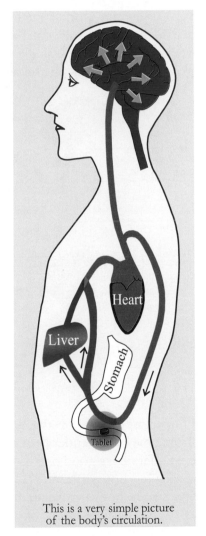

This is a very simple picture of the body's circulation.

Drugs have to be taken every day because they are constantly cleared by the body.

Each tablet only stops seizures for a short time

Tablets do not work straight away. It usually takes several hours before they are dissolved in the bowels, are taken up by the blood and work in the brain. One single tablet is rarely enough to stop the brain from producing epileptic seizures.

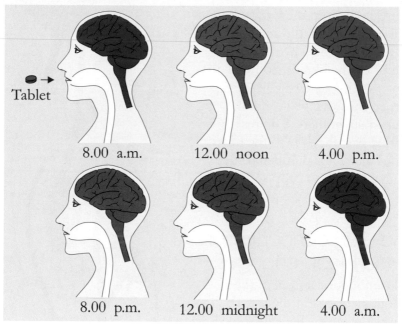

The picture shows how the high risk of a seizure (red) is lowered for a short time by the antiepileptic drug (shown in blue). In this example the tablet offers good protection for about 8 hours. It only begins to work a few hours after the tablet has been swallowed because it takes time for the body to take up the active ingredients and to deliver them to the brain. The effect of the drug wears off because the body breaks it down and clears it.

Some antiepileptic drugs have to be taken several times a day.

Drugs have to be taken regularly so that they can protect against seizures

To achieve protection against seizures around the clock, the same amount of a drug has to be fed into the body as is broken down and passed out. This sort of balance is called "steady state".

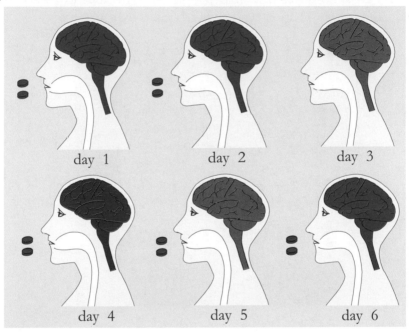

day 1   day 2   day 3

day 4   day 5   day 6

If tablets are taken regularly (for instance as two tablets once a day) and at the right dose, the amount of the drug which enters the body is the same as the amount which passes out of it. The concentration of the drug in the brain (blue) will then remain steady. If tablets are forgotten or drugs are not taken up by the bloodstream because of vomiting or diarrhoea, the risk of seizures (red) goes up as on days 3, 4 and 5.

Tablets have to be taken every day because it is not known when seizures could happen.

A dosette box can make it easier to take tablets regularly every day

If tablets are not taken regularly, the brain is not always protected against seizures. Taking tablets on and off can even make epilepsy worse. Dosette boxes can help people to remember to take their tablets every day. These boxes can hold tablets for a whole week.

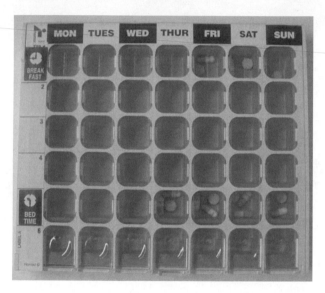

This is a picture of a dosette box for one week. There are several compartments for each day, for the morning, lunchtime, afternoon and so forth. The box can be filled once a week. Each compartment can be opened separately with a slider. The dosette box in the picture has been used up to Thursday afternoon. The Thursday morning tablets have been taken. The owner of the box takes three tablets at night-time.

People with epilepsy who have become free of seizures through antiepileptic drugs should not risk having more seizures by not taking their tablets regularly. As drugs are broken down and cleared by the body all the time, they have to be topped up regularly.

3.3 Antiepileptic drugs

Antiepileptic drugs act on nerve cells in the brain

Many effects which drugs have on nerve cells are known. However, it is often not clear which one of the effects (or which combination of effects) stops seizures. At the moment, only three of four people with epilepsy can be treated successfully with the drugs available. This means that there is a great need for new antiepileptic drugs.

New drugs are often discovered in the way in which Christopher Columbus discovered America 500 years ago. Unlike his contemporaries he thought that the world was not flat but round. So he sailed off to the west to find a new sea route to India. He found America by chance.

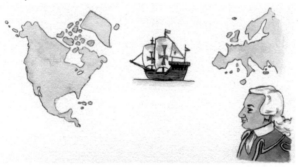

Most antiepileptic drugs were also discovered by chance. For instance, forty years ago, scientists were looking for new drugs for heart conditions. They produced chemical substances which seemed likely to have effects on the heart. However, the substances they had made could not be dissolved in water. Therefore, they could not have reached the heart through the blood. To help dissolve the drugs in water, they were mixed with a substance called dipropylacetate. As it happened, the new drugs had no effects on the heart. However, it was noted by chance that they stopped epileptic seizures. Some time later, the scientists realised that it was not the useless heart drugs which were stopping seizures but the dipropylacetate. Today this substance is used as valproate.

Drugs can stop the development of epileptic activity in the brain

Seizures are caused by abnormal electric tension in nerve cells. In the picture, a nerve cell producing such epileptic activity is marked in red. Research is beginning to explain how epileptic activity develops. Little channels in the wall of the nerve cell play an important role. In particular, channels specialising in the transport of calcium ions and potassium ions are responsible for the development of epileptic activity.

Nerve cell producing epileptic activity whilst being flooded with calcium ions

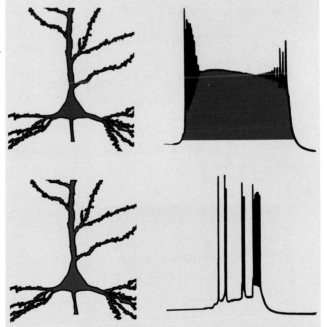

Treated nerve cell, protected from being overwhelmed by calcium ions

Many antiepileptic drugs have an effect on the channels in the cell wall. Drugs which hold up the flow of calcium ions into the cell can stop epileptic activity and seizures. Epileptic activity can also be stopped by blocking the flow of sodium ions or by increasing the flow of potassium ions into cells. Several of the antiepileptic drugs used today work in this way.

Drugs can stop the spread of epileptic activity in the brain

An epileptic focus is an area of the brain which produces epileptic activity. In the picture, the focus is marked red. The brain surrounds such a focus with a rim of cells (marked blue) whose job it is to stop the spread of epileptic activity to the rest of the brain.

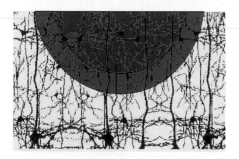

Epileptic focus with rim of brain cells trying to stop the spread of epileptic activity

This rim acts like a dam which stops epileptic activity from spilling over to other brain areas. Antiepileptic drugs can strengthen this rim and help protect the rest of the brain.

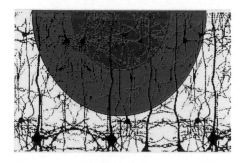

A drug has strengthened the rim around an epileptic focus.

Some drugs do not stop the production of epileptic activity (which can still be seen in the EEG), but they do stop the spread of this activity. They can do this by strengthening the brain's defences against epileptic activity.

Drugs can stop brain cells from falling in step with one another

The epileptic signals which are picked up in the EEG and which cause the twitching of muscles during a seizure are produced by groups of nerve cells firing off electric tension in step with one another (or synchronously). This sort of "synchronicity" is typical of epileptic activity and means that many nerve cells are firing at the same time. The picture shows a group of nerve cells producing abnormally synchronous epileptic activity.

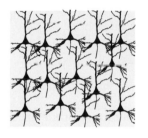

Without an anti-epileptic drug

All cells suddenly produce epileptic activity in step with one another.

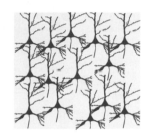

Seizures can be prevented by stopping groups of brain cells from discharging electric tension at the same time. Drugs acting in this way would stop epileptic activity in the EEG.

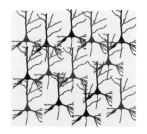

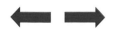

After treatment with an antiepileptic drug

Cells do not discharge at the same time.

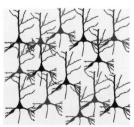

Several epilepsy drugs can affect groups of nerve cells in this way. They act by different chemical means and may work on different centres in the brain.

Carbamazepine (CBZ)

Carbamazepine (CBZ) is one of the most commonly used antiepileptic drugs. CBZ is the name of the active substance (the generic name). CBZ is contained in the protected brands Carpaz, Degranol, Epimaz, Mezipine, Novo-Carbamaz, Prozine, Tegretol, Temporol, Teril, Timonil (not all of which are available in the UK). Some brands are additionally marked "MR" (modified release) or "retard". Such tablets release CBZ more slowly in the body.

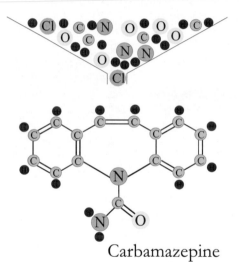

Carbamazepine

The drug is made up of:

Ⓒ : Carbon
● : Hydrogen
Ⓝ : Nitrogen
Ⓞ : Oxygen

Like most other drugs, CBZ is broken down and passed out by the body all the time. Tablets therefore have to be taken at least twice a day.

Carbamazepine dissolves in the intestine and is taken up by the bloodstream. It is broken down in the liver. If seizures were first stopped by carbamazepine and then started again, the amount of CBZ in the body may have dropped. The amount of CBZ in the body can be measured with a blood test. Sometimes a higher dose can stop seizures again. In other cases, a different antiepileptic drug or a combination of drugs would be better.

CBZ can stop seizures without removing the typical epileptic signals from the EEG. Such EEG-signals suggest that the normal working of the brain can still be disturbed even if there are no further seizures.

Carbamazepine is often used as the first antiepileptic drug. It can stop many types of seizures. However, one can never be certain which dose will stop the seizures. As with other antiepileptic drugs, the right dose has to be found for everyone. People who have never been treated with antiepileptic drugs before often become free of seizures with a very small amount of CBZ.

CBZ often does not work for absence seizures, it may even make them worse.

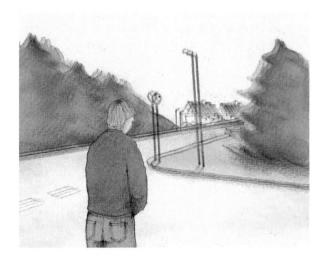

Occasionally, carbamazepine causes side-effects. Some people have an allergic reaction to it. Usually this causes a skin rash. Most people who are allergic to CBZ have to stop taking it.

Double or blurred vision is a common side-effect of CBZ. It is not dangerous unless people are doing something for which they need clear vision. The double vision always settles when the amount of CBZ is reduced. However, changes of antiepileptic drugs should always be discussed with a doctor first.

CBZ causes the liver to break down other drugs more quickly. This weakens the effects of the oral contraceptive pill. People on CBZ who want to stay on oral contraceptives have to take a double dose of the Pill. They may also consider using other forms of contraception like condoms or a coil.

Phenytoin (PHT)

Phenytoin has been used as a treatment for epileptic seizures for some 70 years. Phenytoin is the name of the active ingredient which is contained in the registered brands Dilantin, Epanutin, and Epamin (not all of which are available in the UK). Apart from PHT tablets, capsules or syrup, there is also a solution of PHT which can be injected into a vein. The capsules or tablets contain 25, 50 or 100mg of PHT. The solution is mostly used in hospital as a treatment for status epilepticus.

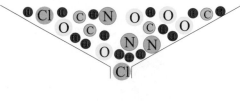

The drug is made up of:

Ⓒ : Carbon
● : Hydrogen
Ⓝ : Nitrogen
ⓞ : Oxygen

Phenytoin is broken down and passed out of the body by the liver. To replace the amount passed out of the body it has to be taken at least once a day.

Phenytoin

Phenytoin is only taken up slowly from the intestine. Because of this the level of PHT rises gradually over 6 hours after a tablet has been taken. After 6 hours the amount of PHT begins to fall and, after around 30 hours, only half the amount of PHT is left in the body. Given that it stays in the body for such a long time, it is possible to take the whole amount of PHT needed to protect the brain for the day in a single dose.

Phenytoin is used for generalised or focal seizures. It does not tend to work very well for seizures in babies or toddlers. Many people get no side-effects from PHT. However, as with other drugs against seizures, side-effects are more likely when people take high doses of PHT. High levels of PHT can cause nausea, vomiting, double vision, dizziness and trembling of the hands.

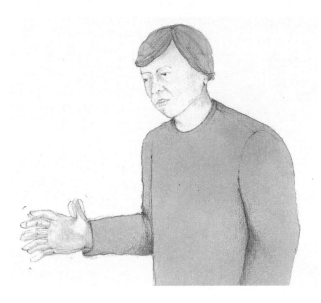

Sometimes, PHT can affect the way people look, for example it can cause the gums to grow thicker. Such thickening of the gums (or gum "hypertrophy") can be corrected. It can also be prevented to some extent by taking good care of the teeth. Rarely, PHT can cause an increase of body hair or brown patches on the skin.

PHT can reduce the effect of other drugs. Drugs that work less well when people also take PHT include blood thinning treatment and the oral contraceptive Pill. Women who need to take PHT and who also want to take the pill may need to take a double dose of the pill.

Valproate (VPA)

Valproate or valproic acid are chemically related to fats. It is the active ingredient in the brands Convulex, Epilim, Orlept, and Valpro (not all of which are available in the UK). The word "Chrono" is added to tablets which contain a form of VPA which lasts longer in the body so that it can be taken once a day. Each tablet contains between 100 and 600mg of VPA. VPA is available as a syrup and a solution for injection into a vein.

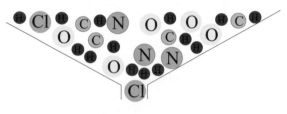

The drug is made up of:

C : Carbon

⬤ : Hydrogen

o : Oxygen

A : Various additions, for instance sodium

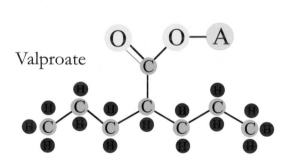

Valproate

Valproate is broken down and passed out of the body by the liver. It has to be replaced once or twice a day.

Normally drugs are stronger if their amount in the body is greater. When treatment with VPA is started, the total amount of VPA in the body increases over some days. Eventually, the amount of VPA taken and the amount passed out every day are in balance. Although the amount of VPA in the body does not increase after this, its effectiveness against seizures continues to grow stronger for some time.

Valproate is often used to stop generalised seizures but it also works for focal seizures. VPA is particularly useful for stopping absence seizures. Seizures which are provoked by flashing light and other primary generalised seizures can also be treated with VPA.

VPA can cause stomach pain and sickness. This can be reduced by using forms of VPA which dissolve slowly in the intestine. Most side-effects caused by valproate occur soon after starting the treatment and pass after a while. Valproate can reduce the ability of the blood to seal off small wounds. Some people who have this problem can bruise easily or can have nose bleeds. People who take VPA should warn a surgeon or a dentist about this before they have an operation.

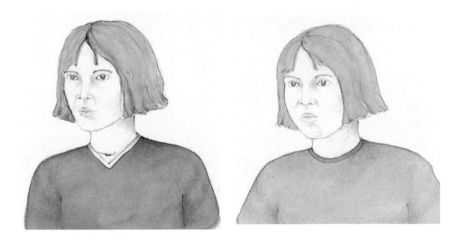

Valproate can also affect people's looks. It can, for instance, cause hair loss. Although the hair usually grows back if VPA is stopped, it sometimes is more crinkly and has a slightly different colour from the original hair. VPA can cause weight gain. This means that people taking VPA should keep an eye on their weight. Women who take valproate can develop irregular periods. Occasionally VPA makes acne worse. Severe damage to the liver can be another (but extremely rare) side-effect of VPA.

Phenobarbital (PB)

Phenobarbital belongs to a group of substances called barbiturates. Phenobarbital is also made by the body when it breaks down primidone, another drug used to treat seizures. PB is contained in the brands Luminal and Gardenal (it is only available as a generic drug in the UK). Apart from tablets, there is a PB syrup and a solution which can be injected into veins or muscles. Barbiturates have been used to treat seizures for about 90 years. In the past, they were also used as sleeping tablets. They are still given today to put people to sleep for operations.

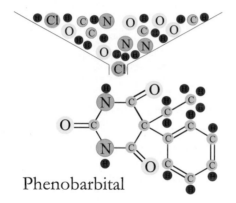

Phenobarbital

The drug is made up of:
C. Carbon
H. Hydrogen
o Oxygen and
N Nitrogen

Phenobarbital is broken down by the body all the time and has to be replaced at least once a day.

Phenobarbital is only taken up slowly in the intestines. It is also broken down and passed out of the body at a slow rate. This means that it is possible to replace the whole amount of PB needed for the day in a single dose. If PB is started at such a replacement or "maintenance" dose, it takes 3 weeks for the drug level to build up in the body. If PB has to be started more quickly, it can be introduced with a higher "loading" dose which is then lowered to the normal daily dose after a few days. If PB is stopped it takes a long time until the drug has passed completely out of the body. PB can reduce the effect of the oral contraceptive pill and it can cause a lack of vitamin D which can weaken the bones .

Phenobarbital is an effective treatment for generalised and focal seizures. It can also be used in status epilepticus. It is sometimes used in small children to prevent seizures with high temperature (febrile convulsions). PB can make absence seizures worse.

The main side-effect of PB is tiredness. This is not surprising as PB produces the effects of a general anaesthetic if it is taken in high doses. In children, PB sometimes causes the opposite effect, overactivity and unusual irritability. PB can also cause difficulties with concentration and it may increase reaction time. This can cause problems if people have to react quickly in traffic or if they operate dangerous machinery.

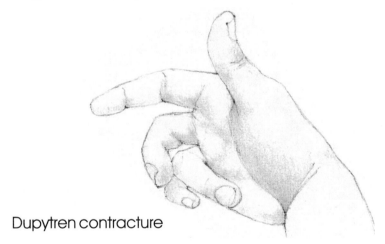

Dupytren contracture

People who have taken Phenobarbital for many years sometimes develop a condition called "polyfibromatosis". There is thickening of the connective tissue, particularly in the hands. The tendons become thicker and shorter, and it becomes increasingly difficult for people to stretch their fingers (Dupytren contracture). The shoulders may be affected, too.

PB should never be stopped suddenly. This can cause "withdrawal" seizures.

Benzodiazepines (BDZ)

Benzodiazepines are a group of drugs. A number of BDZ are used to treat seizures: clobazam, clonazepam, diazepam, lorazepam, midazolam and nitrazepam. The following brands contain benzodiazepines: Frisium, Klonopin, Paxam, Rivotril, Alupram, Antenex, Atensine, Benzopin, Betapam, Calmpose, Dialag, Dialar, Diaquel, Diazemuls, Doval, Ducene, Dynapam, Ethipam, Evacalm, Meval, Novo-Dipam, Pax, Rimapam, Scriptopam, Solis, Stesolid, Tensium, Valclair, Valium, Vivol, Almazine, Ativan, Tranquipam, Mogadon, and Nitrazodon (many of these are not used in the UK). BDZ can be given as tablets, can be injected into a vein, the nose or into the back passage. BDZ are not only used in the treatment of epileptic seizures. They also have many other uses, for instance as sleeping tablets and to help in the treatment of anxiety.

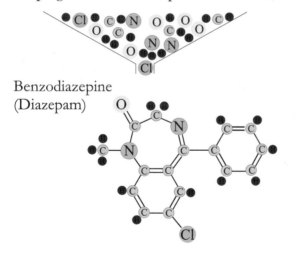

Benzodiazepine
(Diazepam)

The drug is made up of:

Ⓒ : Carbon
● : Hydrogen
Ⓞ : Oxygen
Ⓝ : Nitrogen
Ⓒⓛ : Chloride

Like other drugs, BDZ are broken down and passed out of the body all the time.

BDZ act very quickly and can be injected into a vein or into the back passage during status epilepticus. To inject BDZ into the back passage a "rectiole" is passed into the rectum like a suppository and its content is squirted out. However, it is important not to give too much as this can cause the blood pressure to fall and breathing to stop.

Benzodiazepines work very well for most types of seizures. They can sometimes block seizures which were not stopped by carbamazepine or phenytoin. Unfortunately, the effect of BDZ wears off in most people and then can stop working altogether after a while. When this has happened, they usually work again once they have not been taken for a few weeks. Because of these problems, BDZ are rarely used in the long-term treatment of seizures. However, they are very useful for status epilepticus, or in people who only have seizures at particular times, for instance women who only have seizures around their period.

The main side-effect of BDZ is tiredness and poor concentration. BDZ can affect reaction time and may therefore cause problems when people have to react quickly in traffic or when they operate dangerous machines. In children, BDZ can sometimes cause irritability and hyperactivity.

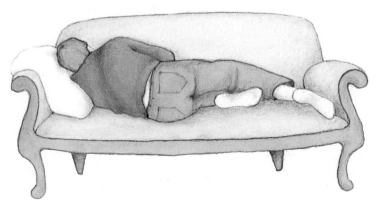

If BDZ are taken for some time, people can become addicted to them. The main symptom of such an addiction is that people who suddenly stop their BDZ feel very anxious. They can also develop muscle cramps or the kind of problems heavy drinkers have when they stop alcohol suddenly. Such withdrawal symptoms are not common in patients who take BDZ for epilepsy. One reason for this is that the BDZ doses used to treat seizures are relatively small.

Lamotrigine (LTG)

Lamotrigine has been used to treat seizures for about twenty years. Lamotrigine is contained in the brand Lamictal. Several studies have shown that LTG is an effective treatment for seizures. LTG was developed to block the effect of folic acid in the body. Folic acid is a vitamin which is found in liver and yeast. Like all other vitamins, the body needs folic acid. However, folic acid can make seizures worse.

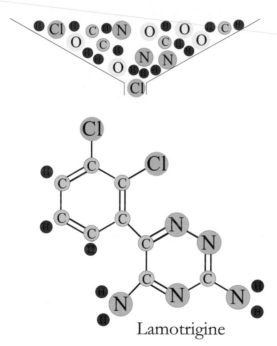

Lamotrigine

The drug is made up of:

Ⓒ : Carbon
● : Hydrogen
Ⓒⱡ : Chloride and
Ⓝ : Nitrogen

Lamotrigine may be used on its own or in combination with other drugs. It can work for generalised and partial seizures. It is broken down and passed out of the body all the time. It has to be replaced at least once a day.

Lamotrigine has a similar effect on seizures as phenytoin and carbamazepine. Sometimes LTG reduces epileptic activity in the EEG without actually reducing the number of seizures. It is possible that the brain works better if it is disturbed less often by epileptic activity but LTG would have to be combined with another drug in such a case to stop seizures.

Lamotrigine can be used on its own (as "monotherapy") or in combination with other drugs. It can stop seizures in many types of epilepsy.

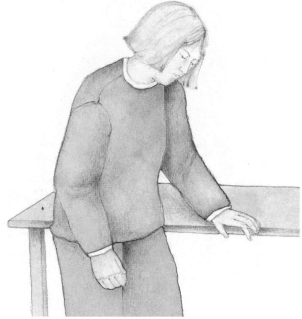

Lamotrigine rarely causes side effects. In higher doses it can cause weakness, tiredness and double vision. About 2% to 3% of people develop an allergic skin reaction to LTG. This can often be prevented if the amount of LTG taken every day is increased very slowly, over several weeks, when treatment is first started. If a skin rash develops, it could be a sign of a serious allergic reaction. It should always be discussed with a doctor. Most skin rashes caused by LTG will disappear quickly if it is stopped or the amount taken every day is reduced.

As a positive side-effect, LTG sometimes improves mood in people who were feeling low. LTG does not affect the action of other drugs (like the contraceptive pill).

Gabapentin (GBP)

Gabapentin is another relatively new drug treatment for seizures. It is contained in the brand Neurontin. GBP was originally designed to imitate the body's own substance GABA, which can suppress seizures. However, its actions on the brain are quite different from those of GABA. It seems to stop seizures by slowing the flow of calcium into nerve cells.

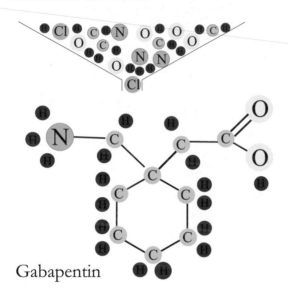

Gabapentin

The drug is made up of:

Ⓒ : Carbon

● : Hydrogen

Ⓞ : Oxygen and

Ⓝ : Nitrogen

Gabapentin is passed out of the body by the kidneys without being broken down. It has to be replaced three times a day.

Gabapentin is quickly taken up by the body and passed out again. After about 7 hours only half the amount taken is still inside the body. Because of this, it is recommended that the drug should be taken three times a day. Gabapentin does not affect the action of other drugs (for instance the contraceptive pill).

Gabapentin rarely causes side-effects. Some people, however, develop tiredness, dizziness, problems with balance or concentration. These side-effects are usually mild and settle after 2 weeks or so if people keep taking the tablets. Very few people have an allergic reaction to Gabapentin.

Oxcarbazepine (OXC)

Oxcarbazepine is chemically related to the drug carbamazepine and it is used in a very similar way. Oxcarbazepine is contained in the brand Trileptal and Timox. Like Carbamazepine OXC may stop seizures by blocking sodium channels in the wall of nerve cells in the brain.

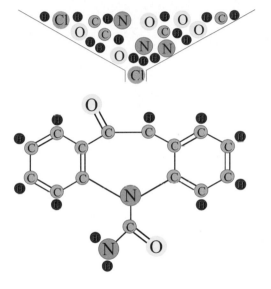

Oxcarbazepine

The drug is made up of:

Ⓒ : Carbon
⬤ : Hydrogen
Ⓝ : Nitrogen and
o : Oxygen

Like other drugs, OXC is broken down and passed out of the body. The amount which is broken down each day has to be replaced each day.

Oxcarbazepine is less likely to cause side-effects than Carbamazepine. Some people may be able to take doses of OXC which would cause side-effects if they were treated with carbamazepine. Although OXC and carbamazepine are chemically similar, they are broken down in different ways. Perhaps this is why OXC causes fewer side effects than carbamazepine. In higher doses, however, OXC can cause the same side-effects as carbamazepine. Some people develop an allergic reaction to OXC. OXC weakens the effect of the contraceptive pill.

Ethosuximide (ESM)

Ethosuximide belongs to a group of drugs called succinimides. ESM is contained in the brands Emeside and Zarontin. ESM is chemically similar to methsuximide which is contained in the brand Celontin, and phensuximide in the brand Milontin. Succinimides have been used for epilepsy for about 50 years. ESM is available in tablet or syrup form.

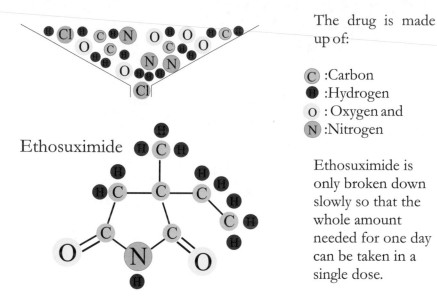

Ethosuximide

The drug is made up of:

ⓒ :Carbon
● :Hydrogen
ⓞ : Oxygen and
Ⓝ :Nitrogen

Ethosuximide is only broken down slowly so that the whole amount needed for one day can be taken in a single dose.

Ethosuximide is mainly used for absence seizures in children and adolescents. It does not stop tonic-clonic seizures. If people also have tonic-clonic seizures, they cannot be treated with ESM alone. ESM is often combined with valproate because these two drugs work very well together.

ESM rarely causes side-effects. If there are side-effects, they are most likely to develop shortly after starting the drug. Very rarely, ESM may cause changes in thinking and anxiety. Like most other antiepileptic drugs, ESM can cause an allergic reaction in some people.

Primidone (PRM)

In chemical terms, primidone is closely related to phenobarbital. The body breaks most of the PRM down to phenobarbital, so the strengths and side-effects of the two drugs are very similar. PRM is contained in the brands Cyral, Lepsiral, Liskantin, Mysoline, and Resimatil.

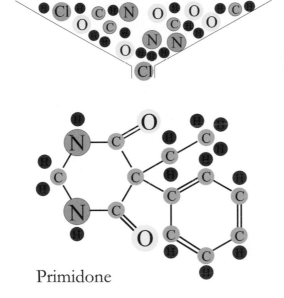

Primidone

The drug is made up of:

- C : Carbon
- ● : Hydrogen
- o : Oxygen and
- N : Nitrogen

Primidone blocks generalised and partial seizures, expecially in adults. It does not tend to work well for complex partial seizures.

As with phenobarbital, the dose of primidone has to be increased and reduced slowly. The amount of PRM should not rise or fall quickly in the blood. This means that it can take weeks or months to stop PRM.

PRM has the same side-effects as phenobarbital, mainly tiredness and problems with concentration. However, some people get nausea or an allergic skin reaction from PRM. Most physicians prefer phenobarbital to primidone.

Levetiracetam (LEV)

Levetiracetam is contained in the Keppra brand of antiepileptic drugs. It is a further development of the drug piracetam which is sometimes used in the treatment of certain myoclonic seizures. In contrast to piracetam, LEV may work for all seizure types, although at the moment it is mainly used for focal seizures.

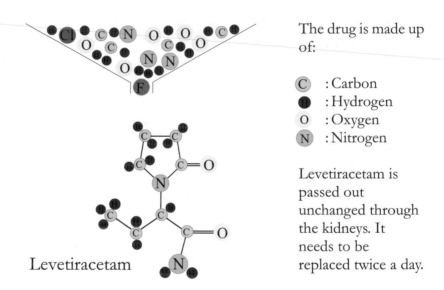

The drug is made up of:

C : Carbon
● : Hydrogen
O : Oxygen
N : Nitrogen

Levetiracetam is passed out unchanged through the kidneys. It needs to be replaced twice a day.

Levetiracetam

Little is known about how levetiracetam works in the brain. It has been shown that it does not act in the same way as any of the other antiepileptic drugs. LEV is usually given in addition to other drugs if they have not stopped seizures on their own. It is so new that there is little experience with LEV on its own. LEV rarely causes side-effects although some people taking it complain of tiredness, difficulty with concentration, nervousness, short temper, or difficulty with sleeping. LEV does not interfere with the action of other tablets in the body and does not change the effectiveness of the oral contraceptive pill.

Pregabalin

Pregabalin is a new antiepileptic drug, which affects the flow of calcium into nerve cells within the brain. It makes nerve cells less able to produce epileptic discharges. Pregabalin is not bound to substances in the blood and does not seem to interact with other antiepileptic drugs. Pregabalin is chemically related to GABA.

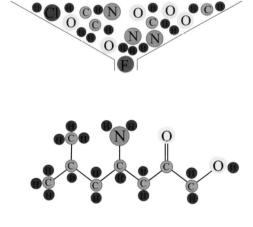

Pregabalin

The drug is made up of:

ⓒ : Carbon
● : Hydrogen
ⓞ : Oxygen
Ⓝ : Nitrogen

Pregabalin is rapidly taken up and passed out of the body essentially unchanged through the kidneys.

Since pregabalin is a new antiepileptic drug it will be tried first as an additional drug if well-known antiepileptic drugs like carbamazepine or phenytoin do not work sufficiently well on their own. Tests have shown that pregabalin is just as effective for focal and secondary generalised seizures as other new antiepileptic drugs. It appears to be ineffective for absence seizures.

Side-effects of pregabalin include drowsiness, tiredness, weight gain and dizziness. Experience with the use of pregabalin is quite limited at present.

Tiagabine (TGB)

Tiagabine is a relatively new drug. It is contained in the brand Gabitril. It is currently only used when another antiepileptic drug (like carbamazepine) does not stop seizures on its own. It is mainly used for focal seizures in the brain.

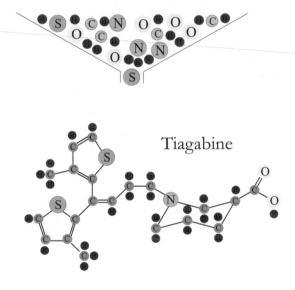

Tiagabine

The drug is made up of:

C : Carbon
● : Hydrogen
O : Oxygen
N : Nitrogen and
S : Sulphur

TGB is broken down and passed out of the body by the liver and kidneys and needs to be replaced at least twice a day.

Tiagabine is quickly broken down and passed out. After six hours only half the amount of TGB taken is still in the body.

Side-effects are commoner in people who take high doses of TGB. Most side-effects come from the brain - dizziness, shakiness, changes in thinking. Sometimes TGB also causes headaches.

Tiagabine was designed to increase the brain's own ability to block seizures. One of the main substances the body uses for this is GABA. Tiagabine is thought to act against seizures by increasing the effects of GABA in the brain. Tiagabine does not reduce the effect of the contraceptive pill.

Topiramate (TPM)

This is a fairly new drug which is contained in the brand Topamax. It can be used in combination with other drugs (like carbamazepine or valproate) or on its own. It is mostly used for focal seizures but it also works for primary generalised seizures.

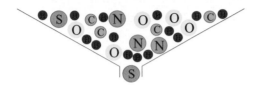

Topiramate

The drug is made up of:

Ⓒ : Carbon
⬤ : Hydrogen
Ⓞ : Oxygen
Ⓝ : Nitrogen and
Ⓢ : Sulphur

TPM is mostly cleared out of the body by the kidneys and needs to be replaced at least twice a day.

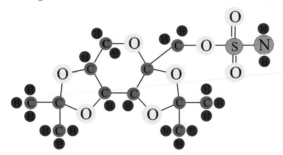

Like many other drugs, topiramate is particularly likely to cause side-effects when it is first started. Most side-effects come from the brain. They include tiredness, dizziness, difficulty with speaking or problems with vision and weight loss. Sometimes people on TPM are more irritable, aggressive or depressed than they were before. TPM can also cause tingling in the face and hands. TPM increases the risk of kidney stones. This risk is smaller if people who take TPM drink plenty of fluid. Topiramate can weaken the effect of the contraceptive pill.

Sulthiame

Sulthiame is the active ingredient in the brand Ospolot. It has been available for over 20 years but it is currently not a licenced treatment of seizures in all countries (it is rarely used in the UK today). Its chemical effects in the body are very similar to those of acetazolamide (brand name Diamox). Sulthiame and acetazolamide affect the dody's ability to control the acidity level in the blood. It is possible that seizures can be stopped by this effect.

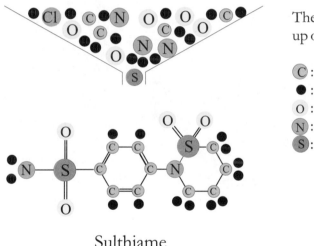

The drug is made up of:

C : Carbon
● : Hydrogen
O : Oxygen and
N : Nitrogen
S : Sulphur

Sulthiame

Sulthiame is a very safe drug which rarely causes side-effects. In Rolandic epilepsy, it reduces the amount of epileptic activity in the brain. Sulthiame is used especially in the treatment of children and adolescents with Rolandic epilepsy. This type of epilepsy is a common form of epilepsy in childhood and affects children between the age of five and ten.

ACTH

ACTH is a hormone made by the body. Its full name is adrenocorticotropic hormone. It is contained in the brand Synacthen. The hormone is made naturally in the brain and is needed to help the body deal with stressful situations. It is a type of protein which cannot be taken in tablet form but has to be injected. We know quite a lot about the effects of the hormone when it is produced in response to stress. However, we do not fully understand why it stops seizures.

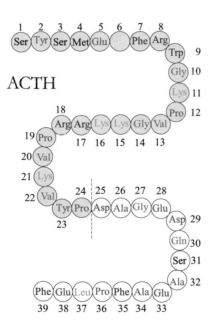

The drug is a protein which is made up of amino acids. Each circle in the diagram stands for one amino acid. The body makes all its proteins out of about 25 different amino acids which can be hooked together in long chains. ACTH is a small protein which only consists of 39 amino acids.

ACTH only works for seizures in small children if a severe type of epilepsy (like West syndrome) cannot be stopped with other drugs. It is a powerful hormone and has to be used with great care. When ACTH has to be given for several weeks, the blood pressure can rise and the body is less able to fight off infections.

Acetazolamide

Acetazolamide is a so-called "second line" antiepileptic drug which can occasionally be helpful. Acetazolamide is contained in the brands Diamox and Novo-Zolamide. The drug is sometimes used when tonic-clonic seizures do not stop (status epilepticus) and when other drugs like benzodiazepines do not work. Acetazolamide is then injected into a vein. The drug is also used in several other diseases like glaucoma and periodic paralysis.

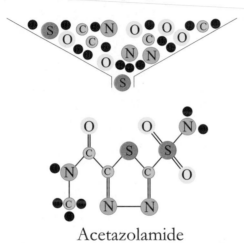

Acetazolamide

The drug is made up of:

Ⓒ : Carbon
⬤ : Hydrogen
ⓞ : Oxygen
Ⓝ : Nitrogen and
Ⓢ : Sulphur

Acetazolamide is rapidly passed out of the body by the kidneys and has to be replaced at least three times a day.

Acetazolamide makes the kidneys pass out potassium. The way it acts against seizures is not fully understood. It causes changes in the blood and nervous tissue which are similar to those seen with the ketogenic diet (which is based on the avoidance of carbohydrates: bread, sweets, vegetables). As with the benzodiazepine group of drugs, the antiepileptic effects of acetazolamide often decrease over several months when it is taken every day. Acetazolamide often causes tingling around the mouth and in the fingers but serious side-effects are rare. It belongs to the chemical group of the sulfonamides (like certain antibiotics). People with known allergic reactions against sulfonamides should avoid acetazolamide.

Zonisamide

Zonisamide is a new antiepileptic drug, which can be added to drugs like carbamazepine or valproate when they do not stop seizures on their own. Zonisamide is contained in the brand Zonegran. Like many other antiepileptic drugs, it was discovered by chance. Zonisamide chemically belongs to the sulfonamides.

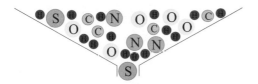

Zonisamide

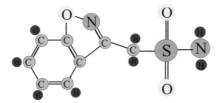

The drug is made up of:

C : Carbon
H : Hydrogen
O : Oxygen
N : Nitrogen and
S : Sulphur

Zonisamide is taken up rapidly but passed out of the body more slowly. It has to be replaced several times a day.

Zonisamide can stop many types of seizures. The way of its action is largely unknown. As with the other drugs against seizures, side-effects appear more often if a greater amount of zonisamide is taken every day. Typical side-effects are drowsiness, tiredness, dizziness and nervousness. Side-effects usually disappear when the amount of the drug in the body is reduced. As with most other new antiepileptic drugs, it is uncertain whether the drug affects the development of babies in the womb.

Felbamate (FBM)

Felbamate is a drug against seizures which is contained in the brand Taloxa. This drug is rarely used although it works against more seizure types than carbamazepine or phenytoin. In fact, it is not licenced as a treatment for epilepsy in the United Kingdom, and has to be imported for individual patients. In particular, treatment with FBM is sometimes considered in people with Lennox-Gastaut syndrome, a form of epilepsy which is very difficult to treat.

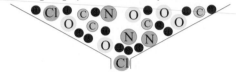

The drug is made up of:

C : Carbon
● : Hydrogen
O : Oxygen and
N : Nitrogen

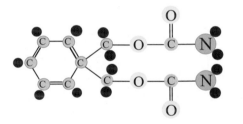

Felbamate

Felbamate is mainly used in children from the age of four and in adults when seizures have not been stopped by

The side-effects of FBM include skin rashes and changes in the blood. The skin rash can be dangerous. It sometimes occurs a few months after the tablets were first started. Small blisters in the mouth are an early sign of this skin rash. The changes in the blood are caused by the body making fewer new blood cells. FBM can also cause liver damage. Because of these possible side-effects, people taking FBM have to have regular blood tests. FBM causes nervousness and irritability when it is taken in large doses.

Vigabatrin (VGB)

Vigabatrin is another antiepileptic drug which has been available for a relatively short time. It is contained in the brand Sabril. Like gabapentin, VGB was designed to imitate the body's own messenger substance GABA, which acts against seizures. The idea was to stop seizures by strengthening the effects of GABA in the brain. It is thought that VGB does this by slowing down the breakdown of GABA in the brain.

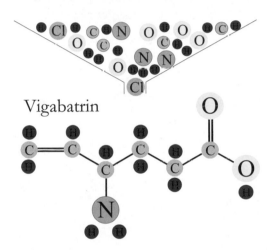

Vigabatrin

The drug is made up of:

Ⓒ : Carbon
⬤ : Hydrogen
Ⓞ : Oxygen and
Ⓝ : Nitrogen

Vigabatrin passes out of the body by the kidneys without being broken down. It needs to be replaced twice a day.

Vigabatrin is sometimes added on to other drugs like carbamazepine. It can be particularly effective against focal seizures which have not been stopped by other antiepileptic drugs. In spite of this advantage, it is not used very often because it damages the visual field in one out of three people. It causes vision to be restricted as if one were permanently looking through a pipe. Vision does not recover when VGB is stopped. In order to detect problems with vision early, people who take VGB should have their field of vision checked regularly. Other side-effects include tiredness and poor concentration. Despite its side-effects, vigabatrin is currently still an important treatment for a type of epilepsy called West syndrome which affects babies and toddlers.

Thiopental and propofol (general anaesthesia)

There is usually no need to interrupt a seizure because most seizures stop on their own. However, if one seizure follows on from another and status epilepticus develops, an ambulance has to be called. In most cases, status epilepticus can be stopped with benzodiazepines like lorazepam or diazepam. When these drugs do not work, phenytoin or phenobarbital are usually given next. However, these drugs may also fail to stop status. If this happens, people are put to sleep as if they were having an operation.

Thiopental   Propofol

The drugs most commonly used to put people in status epilepticus to sleep are thiopental and propofol. Thiopental is a barbiturate drug like phenobarbital but it is given straight into a vein. Like thiopental, propofol is usually used in the operating theatre for general anaesthetics. Once people have been put to sleep with these drugs, normal body functions like breathing, blood pressure and the production of urine in the kidneys have to be monitored closely. Because of this, people requiring these treatments are taken to an intensive care unit and attached to many machines. When general anaesthesia is used to stop status epilepticus, people are usually kept asleep for one or two days.

There are other old and new antiepileptic drugs

Chlormethiazol

Chlormethiazol is contained in the brand Hemineverin. Apart from its effects against seizures it can calm people down and be used as a sedative. It is occasionally used to stop status epilepticus if other drugs (like benzodiazepines or barbiturates) do not work.

Fosphenytoin

Fosphenytoin is a drug which can only be injected into a vein. It is quickly converted by the body into phenytoin. It is only used for status epilepticus or in people who cannot take phenytoin by mouth. It acts more quickly than phenytoin and causes less irritation to veins.

Piracetam

Piracetam is contained in the brand Nootropil. It is sometimes used in the treatment of myoclonic seizures. It is available in tablet form or as a syrup. It is not clear how piracetam stops seizures.

Stiripentol

Stiripentol is another new drug against seizures which is undergoing clinical tests. At present it is not generally available in the UK.

Paraldehyde

The drug paraldehyde has been used against seizures for over one hundred years. It is contained in the brand Paral. Today it is used only for status epilepticus of tonic-clonic seizures. The drug is difficult to handle because light and air break it down and because it is affected by contact with plastic (as in syringes).

Bromides

Salts of the chemical element bromine have been used as antiepileptic drug for about 150 years. Since dangerous side-effects and even poisoning are common, bromides are only used very rarely today.

Many new antiepileptic drugs are being developed

When new substances have been developed, they have to be tried out. The picture shows a test protocol of a group of new substances with possible effects on epileptic seizures.

Substance	Effect	Substance	Effect	Substance	Effect	Substance	Effect
1	-	10	0	19	-	28	-
2	-	11	0	20	-	29	0
3	0	12	-	21	++	30	0
4	-	13	-	22	+	31	0
5	0	14	-	23	-	32	+
6	+	15	0	24	0	33	-
7	-	16	0	25	0	34	-
8	-	17	-	26	0	35	0
9	-	18	-	27	-	36	0
Explanation: - = brings on epileptic activity; 0= no effect; += weak effect on epileptic activity; ++=strong effect on epileptic activity							

Nervous tissue from a snail was treated with the new substances 1 to 36 to see how these substances would affect epileptic activity. The tests show that most of the substances increase epileptic activity or have no effect on it. Only substance number 21 has a strong action against epileptic activity. Further tests have to be performed to check that this substance is not poisonous, for instance on the heart or for a baby in the womb. Substance number 21 can only be given to humans once it has proven safe in many further tests.

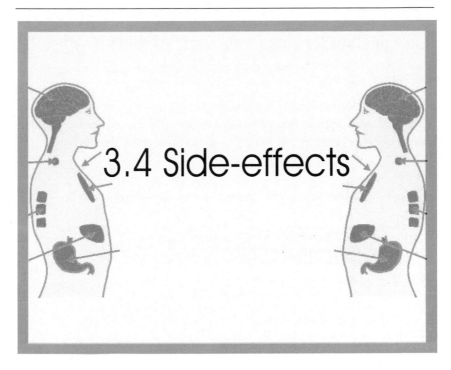

3.4 Side-effects

Drugs should stop seizures; all other effects are side-effects

Many antiepileptic drugs slow people down in their thinking or make them feel tired. Antiepileptic drugs are not given to make people feel less anxious or make them sleepy so these effects are side-effects.

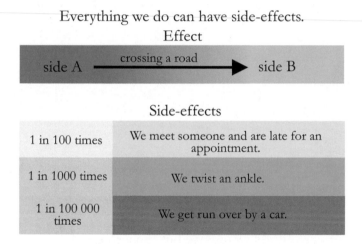

Everything we do can have side-effects.

Effect

side A — crossing a road → side B

Side-effects

1 in 100 times	We meet someone and are late for an appointment.
1 in 1000 times	We twist an ankle.
1 in 100 000 times	We get run over by a car.

Some antiepileptic drugs cause tiredness or drowsiness more often than others. Whereas these problems are rarely caused by lamotrigine, valproate, carbamazepine or phenytoin, they are common with phenobarbital or primidone. The first question in the process of choosing an antiepileptic drug for a particular person is which drugs could stop the seizures. However, other issues are important too - such as which side-effects could develop and what impact they could have on someone's life. Older adults, for instance, may cope better with tiredness than a child going to school. In a woman who might want to have a baby, it is best to choose a drug which would be safe in pregnancy. People who need to take tablets for other medical problems may not be able to take certain antiepileptic drugs.

Side-effects are always a nuisance but can also be dangerous

A particularly nasty and unpleasant side-effect may turn out to be relatively harmless, whereas a side-effect which was hardly noticed, and did not seem especially troublesome at first, could turn out to be dangerous. How ill someone feels with a side-effect does not always show how dangerous it is. It is best to discuss side-effects with a doctor.

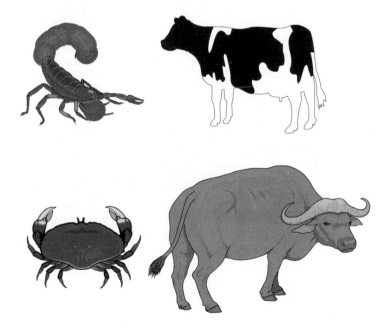

It is often not easy to say how serious a side-effect is based on its first appearance. The same is true of animals. Scorpions look similar to crabs, cows look similar to wild buffaloes. Whilst crabs and cows are fairly harmless, scorpions can be poisonous and wild buffaloes are so dangerous that even lions keep their distance from them.

Treatment should stop seizures without causing side-effects

Many people who go to see a doctor about seizures are worried that antiepileptic drugs are tranquilisers or sedatives given to calm them down. They are often concerned that they could get addicted to them. Some people think that drugs cannot really help with seizures unless they also cause unpleasant side-effects. However, none of this is true.

Reading the drug information sheet often does not help. Information sheets may cause people to worry even more about side-effects.

Drug information sheets contain lists of side-effects. The law says that companies which make drugs have to inform users about any possible side-effect, even if it is rare. This makes it difficult for people who have to take the drugs to judge the actual size of the risk of getting side-effects.

Side-effects are unwanted effects

All drugs can cause side-effects but it is impossible to know who will get them. Some side-effects are more troublesome than others.

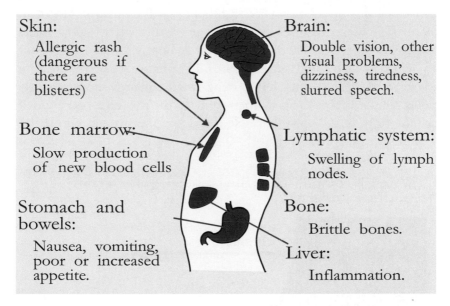

Skin:
Allergic rash (dangerous if there are blisters)

Bone marrow:
Slow production of new blood cells

Stomach and bowels:
Nausea, vomiting, poor or increased appetite.

Brain:
Double vision, other visual problems, dizziness, tiredness, slurred speech.

Lymphatic system:
Swelling of lymph nodes.

Bone:
Brittle bones.

Liver:
Inflammation.

Drugs are taken up by the blood and delivered to the other parts of the body. They are not just taken to the brain but reach all other organs. Mostly, the other organs are not affected by antiepileptic drugs. Sometimes, however, antiepileptic drugs cause reactions like those described in the picture.

Many drug reactions settle with time and are so mild that treatment does not have to be changed. Other reactions may be troublesome but less risky or unpleasant than seizures so that people put up with them. However, there are some drug reactions which are dangerous. In such cases the drug usually has to be stopped, or people have to take a smaller dose.

Side-effects should be discussed with a doctor.

Antiepileptic drugs can cause seizures

Antiepileptic drugs can sometimes cause seizures because each substance acts on the brain in a number of different ways. The main effect will make seizures less likely but other effects may make seizures worse. Usually, the protection against seizures cancels out any effects which could cause seizures. The picture shows that, during weeks 1 to 4, the antiepileptic drug stops seizures more strongly (blue) than it makes them happen (red). If the two effects are added up, the drug is beneficial because it reduces the overall number of seizures the person has.

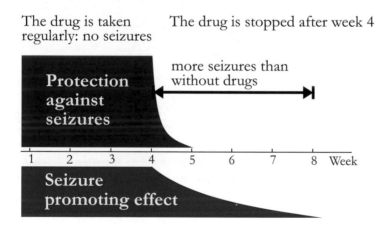

In this example, the antiepileptic drug is stopped suddenly after 4 weeks. The protection against seizures (blue) disappears more quickly than the effects of the drug which may cause seizures (red). In the 5th and 6th week only the seizure promoting effect is left, so that it is likely that more seizures will occur than if no drug had been taken. Stopping antiepileptic drugs suddenly can cause status epilepticus. This is a very dangerous condition in which one seizure is followed by another before the person has fully recovered.

The dose of antiepileptic drugs should only be lowered slowly

The dose of an antiepileptic drug may have to be lowered because of side-effects. If these are severe, and a drug has to be stopped suddenly, seizures can be prevented by another drug which works quickly. However, the risk of an increase of seizures or of status epilepticus is much lower if drugs can be reduced slowly. If possible, antiepileptic drugs should therefore always be tapered off and never stopped suddenly.

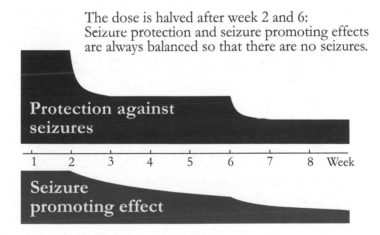

The dose is halved after week 2 and 6:
Seizure protection and seizure promoting effects are always balanced so that there are no seizures.

The diagram shows that the overall effect of antiepileptic drugs is to stop seizures if the dose is reduced slowly (in the example, the total dose is halved two times). Antiepileptic drugs should be stopped slowly because stopping them quickly can cause seizures. They should be started slowly because starting them quickly can cause side-

If antiepileptic drugs are taken regularly, as they are prescribed, they only very rarely cause seizures.

Antiepileptic drugs can change the effects of other medications

Antiepileptic drugs can weaken or strengthen the effects of other tablets. The oral contraceptive pill, for instance, contains hormones which ensure that women cannot become pregnant. These hormones (like many drugs against seizures) are broken down and passed out of the body by the liver.

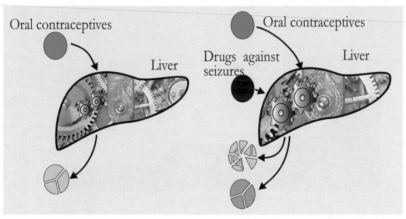

If women take oral contraceptives and antiepileptic drugs, the antiepileptic drugs can cause the machinery in the liver to work more quickly. The body uses this machinery to break down drugs including oral contraceptives (shown in green) and antiepileptic drugs (shown in blue). This means that oral contraceptives are broken down and passed out of the body more quickly. They are therefore less effective and the risk of pregnancy increases. Women who wish to take oral contraceptives together with antiepileptic drugs either have to take a higher dose of hormones to stop pregnancy, or switch to a type of antiepileptic drug which does not make the liver work more quickly. They should discuss this with their doctor.

Antiepileptic drugs can reduce the effect of the oral contraceptive pill.

Antiepileptic drugs can change the effects of alcohol

There is a complicated relationship between alcohol, epileptic seizures and antiepileptic drugs. Most people with epilepsy may drink one or two glasses of beer or wine without any bad effects. However, it is dangerous for them to drink a large amount of alcohol. This can cause an increase in seizures. People who are addicted to alcohol may be at particular risk of this because drinking alcohol can make it harder for them to remember to take their antiepileptic drugs regularly.

Alcohol addiction also puts people at risk of alcohol withdrawal seizures and status epilepticus. Anyone who has to take antiepileptic drugs and wants to drink alcohol has to remember that alcohol increases side-effects so that they may feel drunk very quickly.

Antiepileptic drugs can also increase the effects of other drugs. This may be helpful when a combination of antiepileptic drugs is used to treat people with particularly difficult epilepsy. However, it may also be an unwanted effect, for instance, where antiepileptic drugs increase the effects of tablets for heart conditions. Other tablets can also increase the effects or side-effects of antiepileptic drugs. Because of this, it is important to tell doctors about all current drug treatments before new medication is started.

It is best only to take drugs which are really necessary.

If there are side-effects, treatment should be checked

People with epilepsy should not be afraid to tell their doctor about any concerns they have about their treatment and possible side-effects.

If there are side-effects, several questions need to be answered:

 ## Are the side-effects dangerous?

Side-effects are only rarely so dangerous that treatment has to be stopped immediately. In such cases, people may have to stay in hospital because there can be more seizures or even status epilepticus.

 ## Would the side-effects settle with time if the treatment was continued?

Some people are particularly sensitive to certain drugs, but their body may get used to them. Side-effects which are noticed in the first weeks or months of treatment can settle in such cases. However, people may also be allergic to drugs. It is impossible to predict who will develop an allergy and who won't. Most allergic reactions show up as a skin rash which may be itchy. If the reaction is bad, it may also cause fever. When drug allergies are dangerous they usually affect the inside of the mouth and they cause blisters on the skin. In most cases, allergies are not related to the amount of the drug taken every day.

 ## Is the dose too high?

Many side-effects settle if the dose of the tablets can be reduced. The antiepileptic drug dose which will cause side-effects varies a lot from one person to another. The level at which side-effects occur cannot be predicted. "Dose-related" side-effects include dizziness, tiredness and poor vision (blurred vision or double vision). People may also feel that their thinking is slow. In high doses, most antiepileptic drugs can cause nausea and vomiting.

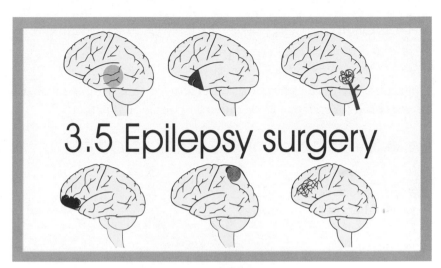

3.5 Epilepsy surgery

In epilepsy surgery, a part of the brain is removed

Operations are never without risk. Because of this, people only have an operation for epilepsy, if a number of conditions are met.

Epilepsy surgery can be considered if...

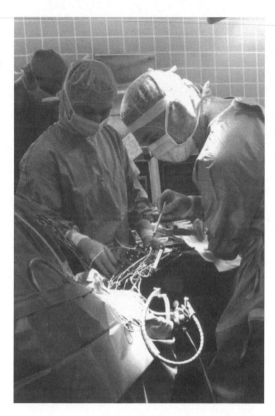

● seizures are so severe that they badly affect people's quality of life.

● a number of antiepileptic drugs have been tried but seizures have continued.

● seizures can only be stopped by using antiepileptic drugs in doses causing troublesome side-effects.

It is never easy to decide whether to go ahead with epilepsy surgery. People considering surgery always have to go through a lot of tests. Some of these tests are not without risk.

Where do seizures start in the brain?

Sometimes, the seizure type suggests where seizures are likely to start. If seizures always start with flashes of light for instance, it is likely that epileptic activity spreads from the vision centre of the brain. If seizures begin with a sudden memory from the past, they are likely to come from the memory centres of the brain in the temporal lobes.

The EEG can help to find the source of seizures

To find out which part of the brain epileptic activity comes from, seizures have to be observed with an EEG. This means that people may have to be attached to an EEG machine for several days. To make seizures more likely during such a recording, antiepileptic drugs may be stopped.

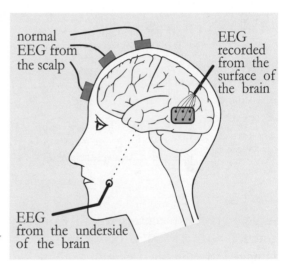

normal EEG from the scalp

EEG recorded from the surface of the brain

EEG from the underside of the brain

In some cases, the EEG has to be recorded straight from the surface of the brain rather than the scalp. To do this, holes have to be drilled into the head and wires are pushed onto the surface of the brain. Sometimes the EEG is also recorded from the the underside of the brain using wires inserted through the cheeks. Recording the EEG from the surface of the brain involves an operation which is not without risk.

For epilepsy surgery, it is important to be certain where exactly seizures start in the brain.

MRI pictures can show where seizures start

Often MRI (Magnetic Resonance Imaging) pictures provide some hint about the source of seizures within the brain. The MRI may, for instance, show changes of the shape or structure of one particular part of the brain. If such changes are seen in an area of the brain in which there are also abnormalities in the EEG, it is likely that seizures come from this part of the brain.

Epilepsy surgery must not disturb the normal working of the brain.

In this picture, the movement, speech and vision centres of the brain are marked in green.

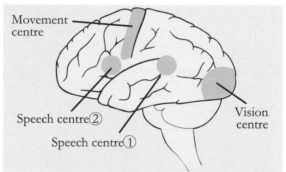

Surgery in these centres would damage one of the important functions of the brain. If, for instance, the speech centre ① was damaged during an operation, there would be problems with understanding the meaning of language. The person affected would hear people talking to him, but he would not understand and he would be unable to answer back. This would be very disabling. One could therefore not consider epilepsy surgery, if the place where seizures came from in the brain was very close to this speech centre.

Some functions are performed by both halves of the brain, so healthy parts of the brain can take over after an operation. Sometimes it is possible to check whether a certain part of the brain is needed for an important function during an operation. This can be done by stimulating the surface of the brain with a small electric current.

Testing functions of the brain can also help to show where seizures start in the brain

The memory for words, for instance, is in an area of the left temporal lobe of the brain. When this area is damaged, the memory for words can work less well. Since seizures start from a damaged area in the brain, a disturbed memory for words can point to the left temporal lobe as the area where seizures start.

By testing brain functions (neuropsychological testing), it is possible to spot an area which is working less well than expected. There are memory tests for words, images or faces, tests for the ability to copy and describe images or to carry out complicated tasks or movements, and tests of the reaction to commands.

Word list read out	Hit, Side, Bark, Shade, Gauge, Pause, Start, Stuff, Mile, Fall
Words learnt initially	Hit, Shade, Pause, Start, Fall
Words remembered after 30 minutes	Hit, Pause, Start, Fall

The diagram shows the result of a memory test for words. The word list at the top was read out several times by the examiner. Immediately afterwards, the person undergoing the test had learnt only 5 of the words. Half an hour later, when he was asked to recall the words again, he could still remember 4 words.

During the test in the diagram, most people learn nine or ten of the words. The poor result of the person in this test shows that there is damage in the part of the brain which deals with memory. The fact that the person tested found it difficult to learn words, but remembered them well later, suggests that the damage is in the outer layer of the left temporal lobe and not in the hippocampus.

The Wada test can prevent damage to the speech centres of the brain

The Wada test (or "intracarotid amobarbital test") is a way of finding out which parts of the brain are important for speech and memory. It is named after Juhn A. Wada, a Japanese epileptologist. The test consists of two steps. At first, the artery which supplies the area of the brain to be examined is inspected by angiography. This is a procedure in which a thin plastic line is put into an artery in the groin and then moved up slowly to the arteries which lead to the brain. Dye, which can be seen on an X-ray machine, is injected to stain up the artery.

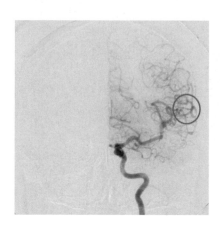

The circle in the picture marks the region which would have to be removed by epilepsy surgery. However, it could contain the speech centre of the brain.

In the second step of the Wada test, the drug amobarbital is injected into the artery. The drug blocks all nerve cells supplied with blood by the artery for a short time. If speech is produced by the area marked in the picture, the person will be unable to speak after the drug injection. This means that surgery would also damage speech.

Two people are counting. In case ① amobarbital has no effect. In case ② speech comes from the marked area in picture.

The person is awake and counts loudly:

① *one two three four five six seven eight nine*
② *one two three fo.. ....*

↓ injection of amobarbital

time →

There is no guarantee that surgery will stop seizures

People who want to have epilepsy surgery have to undergo a lot of tests to ensure that they are likely to benefit from an operation. However, even if the tests go well, there is no guarantee that seizures will stop. Whether seizures stop will only become clear after the operation. Of all people who have epilepsy surgery, only 60% become completely free of seizures. Sometimes it is not possible to cut out the whole epileptic area, sometimes the true source of epileptic seizures in the brain is missed.

When he was six months old, Mr J. had a seizure whilst he was ill with a high temperature. Until he was three years old, he had further seizures when he had fever. When he was 15, he developed attacks which began with an unpleasant sensation in his stomach. Sometimes he would go blank for a minute or two. At 18, he had such an attack but it was followed by a tonic-clonic seizure. Despite taking antiepileptic drugs he continued to have three seizures every week. Mr J. was evaluated for epilepsy surgery. EEG recordings over several days showed that seizures probably started in the left temporal lobe. On MRI pictures, the left temporal lobe looked smaller than the right. To be sure of the source of the seizures, electrodes were placed on the surface of the brain. This showed that seizures came from a part of the brain which was far enough away from the speech centre to consider an operation. During surgery, a part of the left temporal lobe was removed. Mr J. became free of seizures. However, he still has to take antiepileptic drugs.

Whether people benefit from epilepsy surgery depends on the type and cause of seizures, and where seizures come from in the brain.

Epilepsy surgery is mostly performed on the temporal lobes

Seizures which do not stop with antiepileptic drugs often start in the temporal lobes. Compared to other parts of the brain, the temporal lobes are relatively easy to study with tests. This means that it is less difficult to evaluate people with temporal lobe epilepsy for epilepsy surgery.

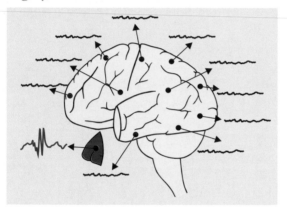

The picture shows that epileptic EEG signals come from the tip of the temporal lobe (also known as the "temporal pole"). Everywhere else, the EEG is normal.

The part of the brain which will be taken away at epilepsy surgery is shown in red. In most operations on the temporal lobe the hippocampus is removed because seizures often come from there. In some people, seizures stop if only the hippocampus is taken out.

Epileptic activity can be caused by all kinds of changes in the brain.

The list of changes in the brain which can cause epilepsy is long. It includes scars, brain tumours, poorly formed brain tissue or blood vessels. If the changes can be taken away, seizures often stop. Sometimes surgery is not just performed to stop seizures but to remove dangerous changes (like tumours or weak blood vessels). In such cases the changes can often be seen so clearly on scans or even with the naked eye during an operation that few tests are necessary before surgery.

Epilepsy surgery in children often involves taking out poorly formed parts of the brain

Some children develop seizures which affect one half of the body. These seizures are often difficult to treat with antiepileptic drugs. The seizures are caused by severe changes in the opposite half of the brain. The changes may have been caused by poor development of the brain or by inflammation. In many cases the arm and leg on the side of the body which is involved in the seizures are stiff, weak or clumsy between seizures.

The striped area in the picture shows the part of the brain which is removed or separated from the rest of the brain during a "hemispherectomy".

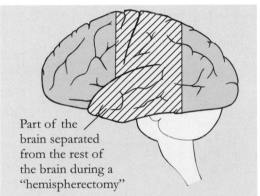

Part of the brain separated from the rest of the brain during a "hemispherectomy"

In most cases it is not known what caused the poor development or the inflammation of a part of the brain. However, it is clear that the damaged parts of the brain can stop the healthy parts of the brain from working normally. Children with severe changes in one half of their brain often do not develop well. They may even lose skills they had before they developed epilepsy. If a "hemispherectomy" can be performed, 80% of these children become free of seizures. They may also become more certain in their movements and able to learn much better. The improvement is often very remarkable. Children can recover lost skills much better than adults.

Surgery works best in children who are younger, and who have not had seizures for long.

A "callosotomy" involves cutting some of the wiring within the brain

Rarely, an epileptic area in one half of the brain can irritate a second area in the opposite half of the brain. Epileptic activity can then spread from there to the rest of the brain. The picture shows how epileptic activity first spreads from A to B and then to the whole brain. Seizures spreading in this way can sometimes be improved by cutting the nerve fibres connecting A and B. However, such operations rarely stop seizures altogether. Sometimes seizures decrease at first but then return over the months and years following surgery.

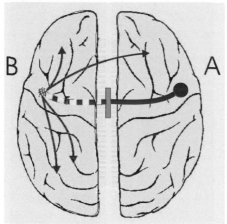

During a "callosotomy" some of the nerve fibres connecting the left and the right half of the brain are cut. The place where this cut is made is marked in blue. Once the cut has been made, the epileptic area in the right half of the brain cannot stimulate the area in the left half. This stops the seizure from becoming generalised.

Mr G. underwent a callosotomy 50 years ago, when epilepsy surgery first started. At this time, the nerve fibres connecting the right half of the brain with the left were sometimes cut completely. The operation improved Mr G.'s seizures but afterwards, the left half of Mr G.'s brain did not always "know" what the right half was up to. With his eyes closed, for instance, he was unable to name things which he was holding in his left hand (because feeling with the left hand is dealt with in the right half of the brain whereas naming things is dealt with in the left half).

Epilepsy surgery is usually offered when there is a good chance of stopping seizures

Operations are most successful when seizures come from changes in the brain which can be seen on pictures of the brain, and which can be removed completely. The removal of abnormal brain cells does not cause problems with the normal working of the brain. Since epileptic tissue can disturb the working of the normal brain cells around it, epilepsy surgery may even improve brain function.

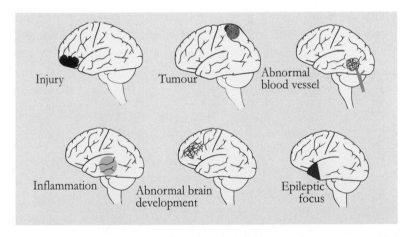

Injury   Tumour   Abnormal blood vessel

Inflammation   Abnormal brain development   Epileptic focus

One of the drawbacks of epilepsy surgery is that once a part of the brain has been removed, it cannot be put back. In most operations, some healthy brain tissue is removed together with the epileptic area. Sometimes this causes problems with the normal working of the brain. The risk of losing functions like memory or speech is reduced by tests before surgery but it is still there. Also, there may be complications of surgery, such as unexpected bleeding or infection. Lastly, the epileptic focus may not be removed completely during the operation, so that seizures may continue after surgery.

A decision about epilepsy surgery is based on many factors.

Surgery using radiation: the "gamma knife"

The gamma knife is a medical instrument, which simultaneously sends out over 200 beams of radiation. The beams enter the brain from different directions, but they are focused on one small target area in the centre. Each individual beam is weak but the radiation is strong where all the beams meet in the brain. It is not clear what exactly happens to nerve cells which have been hit by the radiation. It seems that their metabolism changes.

Just like conventional surgery, gamma knife treatment for epilepsy is only considered after carefully weighing up the advantages and disadvantages for each individual person. Gamma knife treatment can only succeed if the place where seizures come from in the brain is

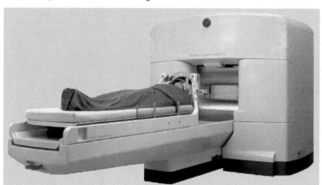

known. The target for radiation is usually identified using magnetic resonance imaging.

Treatment usually consists of a single session of radiation. After this treatment, seizures diminish slowly over the course of a year or so. The treatment itself takes only around half an hour. After this, people are observed in hospital because they can develop swelling of the brain (oedema) which may need to be treated with drugs. One or two weeks later people can return to their usual daily activities. Gamma knife treatment seems to be particularly useful when epileptic seizures are caused by abnormal blood vessels. However, experience with the use of the gamma knife is still limited and little is known about the long term effects of this form of radiotherapy.

Interruption of nerve fibres by "subpial transsections"

The "pia mater" is the soft inner layer of the lining of the brain. Sometimes epilepsy surgery involves making small cuts ("transsections") in the surface of the brain, just underneath the pia mater ("subpial"). Such transsections are performed when the area of brain where seizures start cannot be taken out completely. For instance, if epileptic activity started in the speech areas of the brain, the production or understanding of speech would be damaged if the epileptic focus was removed.

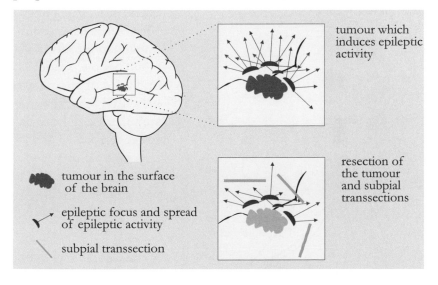

tumour which induces epileptic activity

tumour in the surface of the brain

epileptic focus and spread of epileptic activity

subpial transsection

resection of the tumour and subpial transsections

Transsections can help the brain to block epileptic seizures because epileptic activity spreads through nerve fibres which run along the surface of the brain. Important brain functions like speech or movement, however, rely mainly on nerve fibres, which connect the surface with the central parts of the brain. In many ways, the surface of the brain (the cortex) acts like a screen on which a picture of the world is projected from the inside. Small cuts in the screen would not interfere much with the projected picture.

Epilepsy can also be treated with the electric stimulation of the "vagal nerve"

To do this, an electric stimulator (which works like a pacemaker for the heart) is inserted under the skin. The machine is linked to the "vagal nerve" in the neck with metal wires. This nerve normally carries information from the brain to the organs in the chest and stomach and information from the organs to the brain. The electric impulses from the stimulator are carried into the brain. These impulses affect the nerve cells of the brain so that there may be fewer seizures.

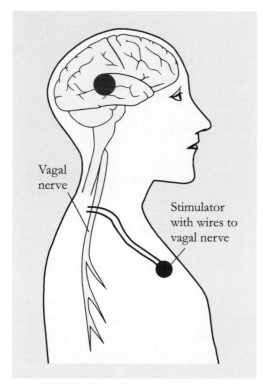

Vagal nerve

Stimulator with wires to vagal nerve

Worldwide, vagal nerve stimulators have been implanted into over 6,000 people. About one third of them have benefited from the stimulator and have had fewer seizures. There may only be two seizures during a period when there would previously have been four attacks.

Some people feel better in themselves with a stimulator in place. It can take up to one year until the full effect of vagal nerve stimulation is seen.

Vagal nerve stimulation can reduce the number of seizures but rarely stops them.

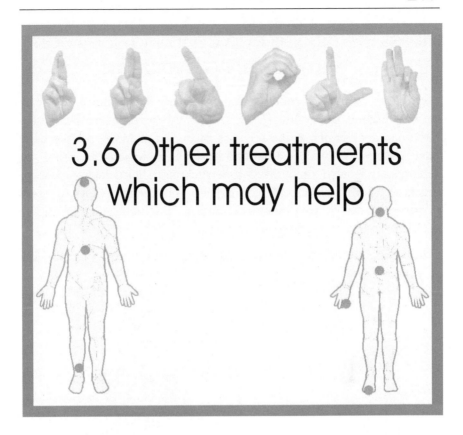

3.6 Other treatments which may help

If seizure triggers can be found, they can sometimes be avoided

Sometimes taking antiepileptic drugs regularly is not enough. It can be worthwhile to try and work out whether there are particular circumstances which make seizures more likely. Many people who have epilepsy know of situations or feelings which can bring on seizures. It is well recognised that flickering light, lack of sleep, drinking too much alcohol or certain moods can help to start seizures. However, the particular situations in which seizures happen are different from one person to another.

Often people feel low, drained or unusually tired before one of their seizures.

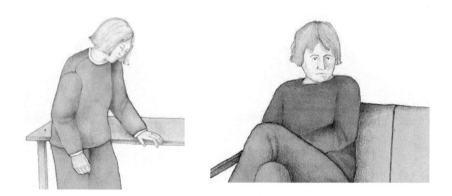

Some trigger factors do not always lead to seizures and are therefore harder to spot. A seizure diary can help to find out about situations in which seizures often happen. Sometimes such situations can be avoided so that seizures are prevented. If this works well and for a long time it may even be possible to reduce or stop antiepileptic drugs. On the other hand, people should not stop doing everything they enjoy out of fear that it may cause a seizure. Some people may prefer higher doses of antiepileptic drugs so that they can continue to do all the things they enjoy doing.

Some people can learn to influence the activity of their nerve cells

During a seizure warning or aura, epileptic activity spreads from the damaged nerve cells which first start the seizure to nerve cells which are otherwise healthy. It is sometimes possible to keep these healthy cells busy with something else so that they cannot become involved in the seizure. This can be done by concentrating on particular images, music or words. People may also try to clench their fist if seizures start there with a tingling sensation. Often people work out how they can stop seizures without any help from others. If a method of stopping seizures has been found, it is important to train the brain by using it every time the warnings of a seizure are felt. This takes a lot of effort and patience.

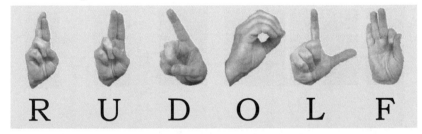

R U D O L F

Often people have to try many different ways of stopping seizures until they find one which works. The person in the picture has learnt to stop seizures by concentrating on spelling the name Rudolf or other words in sign language whenever he feels a seizure coming on. This has reduced the number of seizures quite a lot.

Unfortunately, such methods of stopping seizures only work in very few people. They can only work if there is enough time between the first warning (aura) and the start of the seizure.

Suppressing seizures is hard work, but it can help people who have epileptic seizures with auras.

The EEG can help to stop seizures from developing

The EEG, which shows the electric activity of the brain, can be used to teach some people to suppress their seizures using "biofeedback". In this process a person looks at the monitor of a computer while the EEG is being recorded from their brain and fed into the computer. The computer is progammed to change the picture on the monitor when a certain type of signal is present in the EEG. The person is encouraged to change the picture. In this way, they learn to produce the desired EEG signal. People are then encouraged to produce this particular type of EEG activity on a daily basis.

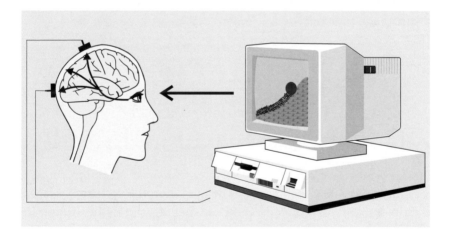

Unfortunately, only very few people with epilepsy can stop their seizures using the biofeedback method. Some people cannot learn how to influence their EEG activity, in other people the method has no effect on seizures.

Some people can stop their seizures by learning the difficult biofeedback method and producing the right EEG-signal.

Desensitisation can help some people with epilepsy

Seizures sometimes happen when people are very excited or stressed. They may be able to avoid such excitement and stress. This may require help from a psychologist or psychotherapist. For instance, if someone is afraid of open spaces which they cannot always avoid, it is possible to reduce anxiety by desensitisation. Desensitisation may be based on the gradual introduction of someone to open spaces which they avoided before. Sometimes seizures disappear together with the person's previous fears.

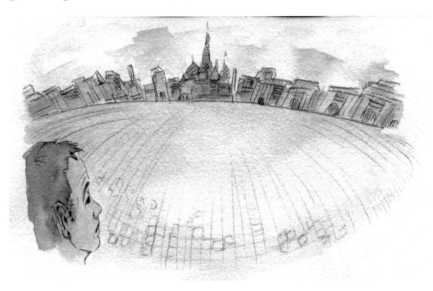

Occasionally, seizures are caused by overbreathing related to anxiety or excitement. Overbreathing leads to a reduction of the carbon dioxide level in the blood. Low carbon dioxide can cause seizures. People can learn to control their breathing so that they do not put themselves at risk of a seizure. They may also be told to breathe back air from a paper bag placed over their mouth. This increases the amount of carbon dioxide in the blood.

Diet can lower the frequency of epileptic seizures

A "ketogenic diet" causes changes in the body's metabolism which make seizures less likely. It is not known exactly how this diet works. It consists of fat and protein. Sugar has to be avoided. Cheese, meat, butter, eggs and oil are good. Bread, cake, sweets, fruit and vegetables have to be reduced or stopped by people trying to follow the rules of the ketogenic diet.

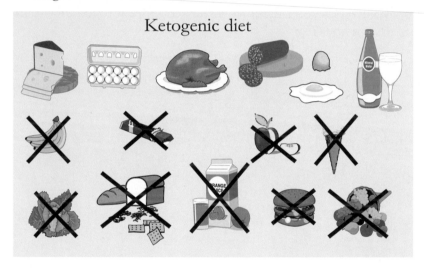

Ketogenic diet

This diet is mainly used in children when antiepileptic drugs have not worked well for severe forms of epilepsy. Its effects start after a few days. Little is known about the long term effects of the diet.

Other diets or diet supplements are sometimes advised for people with epilepsy, but none has ever been proven to reduce the number or the severity of seizures. Some very strict diets should be avoided because they starve people of important nutrients.

Most diets do not work for epilepsy, or seizures come back in the long term.

Sometimes certain smells and tastes can stop seizures

Some people try to find a smell or taste to block the cells which produce epileptic activity in the brain. When they have an aura, they either sniff the smell from a small bottle or they imagine smelling a particular smell. It is important that people take a careful look at whether this approach actually reduces the number of their seizures. They can use their seizure diary for this. Seizures can also be made worse by certain smells.

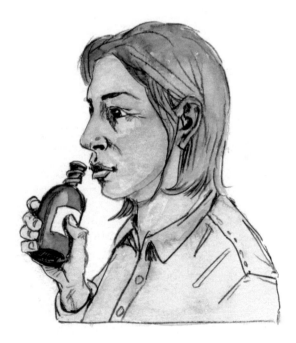

The same smell may stop seizures in one person and cause them in another. Often people can predict whether a particular smell will make their seizures better or worse. Sometimes it is also possible to try to influence seizures through other senses (seeing, hearing, touching).

Acupuncture has not proven successful at stopping seizures

It is not fully understood how acupuncture needles stimulate or calm down the nervous system. Electro-acupuncture uses electricity to stimulate a particular part of the skin. It is easy to imagine that this can stimulate nerve fibres which could have an effect on epileptic activity.

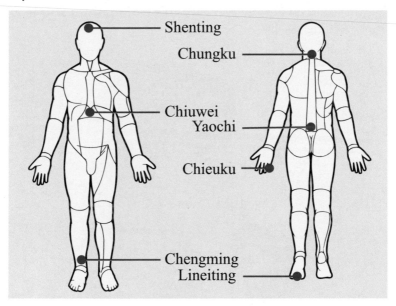

Studies of the effects of acupuncture have not produced clear results. In one study, a group of people with epilepsy was treated by Chinese acupuncture specialists. Only one half of the group were treated with true acupuncture. Stimulation of the true acupuncture points lead to an over 50% reduction of seizures in 39% of the people treated. However 33% of the patients treated with true acupuncture had an over 50% increase of their epileptic seizures.

4 Epilepsy in everyday life

Summary

4.1 Risk and prejudice

Some people are prejudiced about epilepsy. They think that most people with epilepsy have low intelligence, are aggressive or not "normal" in some other way. Many people with epilepsy suffer more because of the prejudice than from the seizures themselves.

It is wrong to make general rules. For instance, it is quite all right for most people with epilepsy to drink moderate amounts of alcohol, or to use computer games, and many people with epilepsy can drive a car. There is no need to ban people with epilepsy from doing sports. In fact, it is a good idea to be involved in sports. However, it is best to take epilepsy into account, and some sports or other activities may not be possible. For instance, people may drown if they have a seizure whilst they are swimming and there is nobody there to help them. People with epilepsy also have to think about their seizures when they are planning to travel. It is best if travel plans are discussed with a doctor. If people with epilepsy want to take part in team sports, it is a good idea to inform other members of the team about the seizures. This gives them the opportunity to ask questions about epilepsy and helps them to react better if they see a seizure. Children and teenagers often find it particularly difficult to tell their friends and teachers about their epilepsy. However, it is often a good idea to try.

4.2 Epilepsy at school and at work

In most cases, people with epilepsy do just as well at school and at work as people without epilepsy. However, their unemployment rate is higher than that of other people. The most important reasons for this are prejudice and the lack of knowledge about epilepsy of the public in general and employers in particular. Over 50% of people with epilepsy complain that life is made difficult for them at their work place. Many choose not to inform their employers about their epilepsy if they have had no seizures for a while. People with active epilepsy may be able to reduce the risk of seizures interfering with their ability to work by choosing a type of work in which the risk to themselves or to others would not be greater than if the seizure happened at home or in public. Most people overestimate the risk of seizure-related injuries at work.

Teachers should know about the types of epilepsy which commonly affect children of school age, and parents should inform teachers of their child's epilepsy. Teachers should know that seizures in the classroom are not their fault, and that they should react to seizures by keeping calm, by ensuring the safety of the child and waiting for the seizure to pass.

4.3 Epilepsy and pregnancy

Getting married or having children are personal decisions which everyone should be free to make for themselves. The great majority of children whose parents have epilepsy or take antiepileptic drugs are perfectly fine. However, the risk of developing epilepsy is slightly increased in such children. If the father or mother has epilepsy, the risk that their child will also develop seizures is about 3% whilst the epilepsy risk in the general population is less than 1%. Antiepileptic drugs taken by the mother can damage babies in the womb. One out of 50 babies born to mothers without epilepsy has a malformation.

However, malformations are seen in four out of 50 babies of mothers taking antiepileptic drugs. The damage occurs most often during the first three months of pregnancy. Because of this, it is a good idea to ask a doctor what can be done to lower the risk of malformations before becoming pregnant. Antiepileptic drugs are contained in breast milk. However the amount is so small that it should not stop women from breast feeding.

4.4 Epilepsy and the law

All men and women are equal before the law. In principle, it is against the law to discriminate against people with epilepsy. However, there are some situations in life in which people with epilepsy are not treated in the same way as people without epilepsy.

People with epilepsy are not allowed to drive if they still have seizures. Once seizures are controlled for at least one year the driving regulations will allow them to drive again. There are special rules for provoked seizures and seizures from sleep.

Another legal problem is whether people with epilepsy are responsible for damage they cause during a seizure. It is extremely rare that a person with epilepsy is considered at fault because of a seizure. They could only be held responsible if the seizure was predictable and avoidable. For instance, a person with epilepsy could be held responsible for damage caused during a seizure in a night club caused by flashing lights - if they knew that the flashing light would trigger their seizures.

There is no general obligation to tell an employer about epilepsy at a job interview. However, people have to be truthful about their epilepsy during an occupational health check. A job offer made before such a health check cannot be withdrawn if the epilepsy would not interfere with the person's ability to do the job in question. There are only a few professions which people with epilepsy cannot take up (for instance working as a train driver or airline pilot). When people develop epilepsy there is an obligation on their employer under the

Disability Discrimination Act to try to enable them to continue in their job. The Employment Medical Advisory Service (EMAS) can help with this.

When dealing with insurance, it is important to be honest about epilepsy. Insurers may not have to settle a claim if they were not told about epilepsy even though insurance premiums may have been paid. Where people already have insurance when they are diagnosed with epilepsy it is important to read the small print. Some insurance companies may need to be informed of significant changes of health status. A new diagnosis of epilepsy would be such a change. Other insurance companies may not need to be told.

4.5 Epilepsy research

Knowledge about epilepsy has grown over hundreds of years. Over the last 200 years, doctors and scientists have published their observations in specialist journals which have helped the science of epileptology to move on more quickly. Advances were often based on new research methods from other fields of science. Today, epilepsy research can be split into basic science and clinical research. Basic science concentrates on nerve cells and their components. It tries to answer questions like: what causes epileptic potentials in nerve cells; which processes lead groups of nerve cells to fall into step with one another; what causes a permanent epileptic focus? Examples of questions asked by clinical researchers are: if drug A does not work, is it better to give drug B or to try drug C; how can we best find the part of the brain where seizures come from; can the EEG be used to predict when seizures will happen? Some of this research is very expensive. Our knowledge about epilepsy would grow more quickly if more money was available for research.

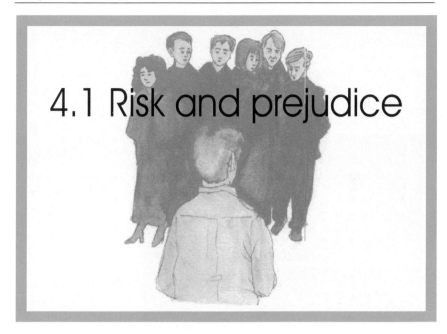

4.1 Risk and prejudice

People with epilepsy can face prejudice

Centuries ago, people with epilepsy were thought to be possessed by demons. The picture shows a priest exorcising the devil from a woman with epilepsy. The devil is flying away in the top left corner.

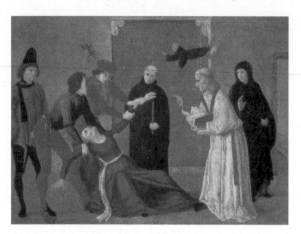

Even today there are things which are said and thought about people with epilepsy that are wrong and can make life difficult for those who have to live with seizures.

The following statements about epilepsy are true.

- People with epilepsy have the same range of intelligence as people without epilepsy.

- Epilepsy does not cause aggression.

- Epilepsy is not a mental illness.

- Most types of epilepsy are not inherited.

The prejudice people with epilepsy face reflects not only how little the general public know about epilepsy, but also the insecurity and anxiety many people feel when they see a seizure. For many, the reaction of others to their epilepsy is worse than the seizures themselves. Rejection and exclusion can cause low self-esteem and low self-confidence.

Having blanket rules for people with epilepsy is wrong

There are many different types of epilepsy and very few rules which could apply to all people with seizures. For instance, contrary to what many people think, all people with epilepsy can watch TV and get involved in sports. If seizures are sometimes triggered by a standard TV, a "flicker-free" set (with a picture frequency of 100 Herz) can help. Seizures can also be avoided by not sitting too closely to the TV set.

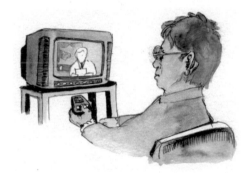

Most people with epilepsy may:

- drink moderate amounts of alcohol;
- go out on their own;
- play computer games;
- drive a car;
- go to night clubs.

Many blanket bans are unnecessary and affect the quality of life of people with epilepsy. Too much alcohol can cause problems with antiepileptic drugs and change the normal daily cycle of waking and sleeping. However one or two glasses of wine or beer hardly ever cause any problems.

Risk should be assessed individually for each person. Everyone needs to discuss the risks which apply to them with their doctor.

People with epilepsy want to lead a normal life

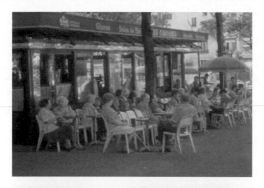

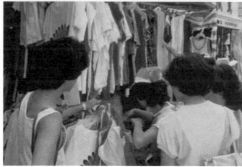

Most people with epilepsy would like to lead a perfectly normal life. However, some may withdraw from others and become isolated because they can face prejudice and feel rejected. The behaviour of others towards people with epilepsy can cause emotional problems like depression. Some people with epilepsy find friendship and support in self-help groups.

People with epilepsy have a normal range of intelligence - just like anyone else.

Some people with epilepsy are highly gifted, others are of average intelligence. In this respect they are no different from people without epilepsy. Because of this, there are children with epilepsy in all types of schools, from A-level colleges to grammar, comprehensive, and special schools. Many people with seizures have completed a university degree and are very successful at work. People who have no health problem other than epilepsy can lead a normal life, both at home and at work, as long as those around them give them a chance to do so.

Sport is fun and can help in difficult times

Sport is fun and gives people the opportunity to enjoy themselves on their own or with others.

It can take the mind off trouble and allows people to let off steam. This may be particularly important for people who have to live with a difficult medical condition.

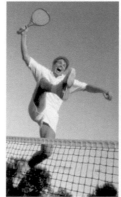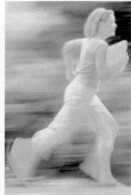

Sports which make people get out of breath do not increase the risk of seizures. Unlike overbreathing for the EEG, increased breathing during sports only helps to provide the body with the oxygen it needs.

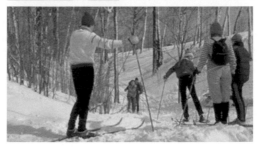

People with epilepsy should not be banned from sports in general.

However, it may be an idea to discuss suitable types of sports with a doctor. Information about sports and leisure activities are also available from organisations like Epilepsy Action and the National Society for Epilepsy.

Most people with epilepsy are able to enjoy sports.

Many people enjoy their sports

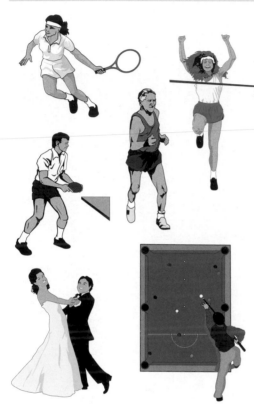

For many people, sport is an important part of life. It helps people to stay fit and healthy and it makes them feel better about themselves. Very few people with epilepsy cannot take part in sports. There is no reason why children with epilepsy should be banned from school sports. Sports clubs can make it easier to mix with others and can help people to feel less isolated. Feeling better about themselves helps people to be more independent and to deal with their seizures. This can improve their quality of life.

The risk associated with sport depends on the type of epilepsy.

In many cases the risk may not be increased at all - for instance if people have enough warning of their seizures to make sure that they are in a safe position or if seizures only happen during sleep. Some people have other problems in addition to epilepsy - like being a little slow or clumsy in their reactions. This should be taken into account when choosing a type of sport.

If in doubt about a sport, it is best to ask a doctor.

The risk also depends on the type of sport

Sports can cause injuries, in people with and without epilepsy. In many types of sport (like badminton, dancing, or table tennis) the risk of injury is no greater for people who have seizures than for those without epilepsy. Other sports are more dangerous, for instance if there is a risk of falling from a height or drowning. In such sports, people with epilepsy may need to be watched carefully by others, take special precautions (like wearing a crash-helmet), or they may be unable to do the sport altogether (like diving or shooting).

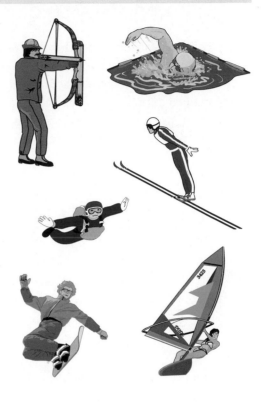

If seizures are likely to happen, it is best to warn team members about them.

This gives them the opportunity to learn about epilepsy and to find out what to do in case of a seizure. Otherwise they may feel helpless and frightened if a seizure happens, and they may not do the right things.

Both the type of sport and the types of seizures should be considered in deciding whether a sport is suitable.

Children with epilepsy develop in the same way as other children

Many children with epilepsy develop normally and do not need any particular support. However, there are some children who do not just have epilepsy but also other disorders of the brain. If children with epilepsy need extra help, it can be difficult to strike the right balance between supporting them and stopping them from becoming more independent. Children who receive too much attention can feel

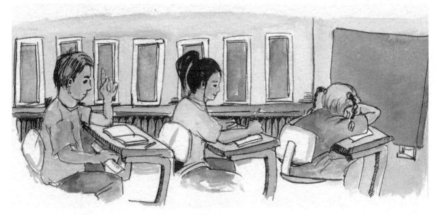

It is not a good idea to let a child's epilepsy take over the life of the whole family. On the other hand, members of the family have to give drugs regularly, help the child when they have seizures, keep a seizure diary, and go to hospital for follow-up visits. It is very difficult to find a middle way between seeming "careless" and being "overbearing". It may help to talk to other parents of children with epilepsy.

Like everybody else, children with epilepsy have to be able to deal with problems and conflicts. They cannot learn this if they are always protected by their families and friends.

Children and teenagers with epilepsy can have a hard time

Young people with epilepsy do not only have to cope with increasing demands from their family and teachers at school, they also have to find ways of living with seizures and their treatment.

Being open about seizures helps teachers, school friends, family members and neighbours to accept a child's epilepsy as part of normal life. Unfortunately, because many people know very little about epilepsy, they may be prejudiced against people who have seizures. Because of this, openness does not always work.

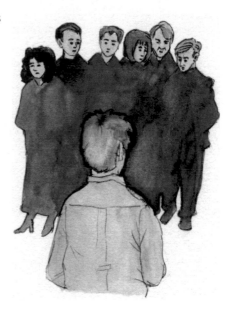

Still, it is generally much better if teachers and school friends know about epilepsy so that they do not get frightened by seizures and know what to do.

Parents of children with epilepsy often have a hard time.

Their child's future may seem uncertain. The child's epilepsy has an impact on many aspects of their lives. Sometimes the stress caused by this leads to friction between the parents. Parents should not hesitate to get advice from other parents of children with epilepsy, from a counsellor or a self-help group if they experience this sort of friction.

Self-help groups help with many family problems.

Many people with epilepsy like to travel

Short trips which do not cause any major changes to the daily routine cause few problems. Longer trips or long distance travel however, need to be planned more carefully. Are vaccinations needed? Is travel going to cause lack of sleep? Is the destination in a different time zone? If so, at what times should tablets be taken? Does the dose of the antiepileptic drugs have to be adjusted? How do you deal with diarrhoea and vomiting if you have to take tablets?

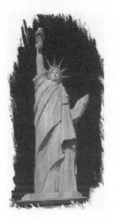 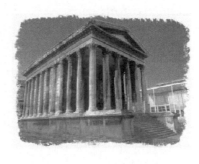

Travellers to some countries need to prepare for their trip by having vaccinations and by taking tablets before they leave to avoid getting diseases like malaria. However, some drugs which are used to prevent malaria are best avoided in people with epilepsy. Travellers to hot countries often develop diarrhoea. Many people treat this sort of diarrhoea with carbon tablets. This is not a good idea for people who have to take antiepileptic drugs as the carbon tablets can reduce their effect. A drug called loperamide is better for diarrhoea in people with epilepsy.

Another thing to think about is health insurance. In most European countries people are covered by the E111 from their post office. In other countries people may need additional travel health insurance.

Longer trips should be discussed with a doctor and planned in advance

Long-distance travel is exhausting and tiring. It can upset the usual daily routine of being awake and being asleep. In some cases, tranquilisers (benzodiazepines) may be helpful. Travelling long distance with the sun (westwards) or against the sun (eastwards) is particularly difficult. Travel in these directions causes days to be unusually long or short. This means that it may be advisable to change the dose of antiepileptic drugs taken on the day of travel. People with epilepsy planning a flight east or west should discuss this with their doctor.

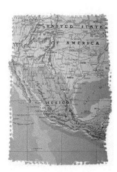

Long-distance air travel, especially to the west or east should be planned in advance.

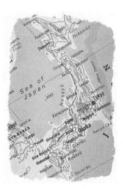

Flying north or south causes fewer problems because this does not affect the normal daily rhythm. Slower modes of travel (like ships) cause less disruption than flying. People travelling by plane should keep all the medication needed for the holiday (and a few extra doses) in their hand luggage, so there is less risk of losing it. A doctor's letter might help to avoid problems at customs.

Extra doses of antiepileptic drugs may have to be taken in case of vomiting or diarrhoea. It is unlikely, for instance, that the body would have taken up much of a drug, if tablets are brought up within half an hour of taking the dose. In this case it may be best to take a second dose. If possible though, advice should be sought from a doctor.

Alcohol can be a problem - for people with and without epilepsy

Alcohol is no problem for people who drink moderate amounts and who do not have to stop themselves from drinking more. However, some people find it difficult to stop drinking. They set out to have one or two drinks but then drink much more. Drinking alcohol can become a dangerous addiction. Often people can only fight this addiction if they stop drinking alcohol altogether. When alcohol addiction is bad, people may need medical help.

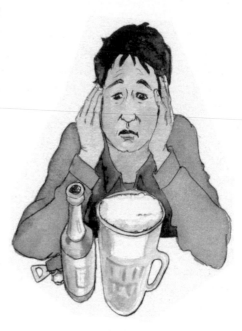

Alcohol can cause epileptic seizures.

Alcohol is broken down in the liver. Whilst drinking, the alcohol level in the blood goes up. Then it falls gradually as the liver clears the alcohol from the blood. Epileptic seizures are particularly likely when the alcohol level in the blood is falling - that is not whilst drinking but afterwards. People addicted to alcohol can develop a degree of brain damage which can cause epileptic seizures. In this sort of epilepsy very small variations of the blood alcohol level may be enough to cause seizures. There is also a high risk of status epilepticus.

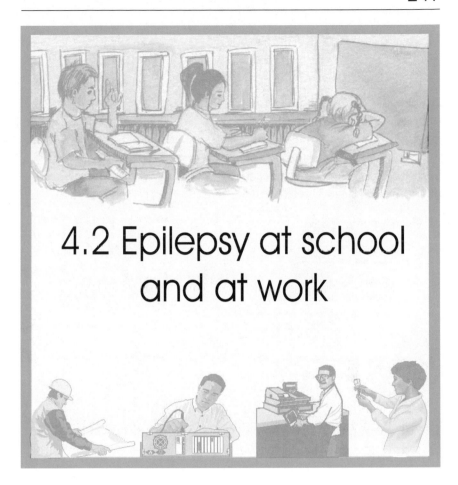

4.2 Epilepsy at school and at work

People with epilepsy can work just as hard as other people

Although most people with epilepsy are keen to work, the unemployment rate of people with epilepsy is higher than that of the general population. Many people with epilepsy are doing low-skilled jobs although they would be able to do more responsible work. This is true despite the fact that people with epilepsy are no more likely to be involved in a work-related accident than others.

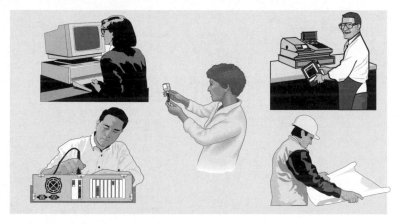

The problems people with epilepsy can face at work are mostly due to prejudice and misunderstanding. Because of this, it is sometimes better not to mention epilepsy when there have been no seizures for a long time. There is no obligation to mention epilepsy at a job interview. However, people have to be honest about epilepsy when they undergo a medical check before they start a job or to find out whether they are able to continue doing their job. A job offer can only be withdrawn or people can only lose their job because of epilepsy, if seizures make it impossible for someone to do their job safely. The Employment Medical Advisory Service of the Health and Safety Executive can offer further advice on this issue.

Many people with epilepsy have unjustified difficulties at work because of epilepsy.

Epilepsy may need to be considered when choosing a career

People who have been free of seizures for many years can do almost any job. A small number of jobs are an exception to this. Even when people have been seizure-free for a number of years they cannot work as lorry or train driver, pilot and soldier. People who are not free of seizures have to consider the risk to themselves and others that come with particular jobs. Jobs which involve using handheld or open machinery could put people at risk of injuring themselves.

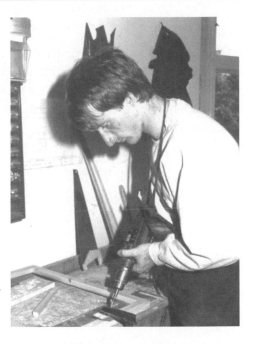

The level of risk also depends on the type of seizures. For example, it would be smaller if someone always had sufficient warning before their seizures to step back from dangerous machinery. If seizures would cause an increased risk of harm to the worker or others, epilepsy should be discussed with the employer. Under the Disability Discrimination Act the employer is obliged to make reasonable adjustments to make the job safe. To do this, they could take advice from the Employment Medical Advisory Service (EMAS). If the workplace cannot be made safe, the employer would be expected to try and find alternative employment in the same company.

The risk of injuries is often over-estimated.

Teachers should be well informed about epilepsy

Often epilepsy is first noticed at school. Teachers should know about three common types of seizures:

Absence seizures: these are brief lapses of consciousness. Children are often thought to be daydreaming at first, and not concentrating on their work. Each absence only lasts a few seconds but one absence attack can quickly be followed by another.

Complex partial seizures: in these seizures, consciousness is often impaired for several minutes. People may seem to behave oddly, they may pick at their clothes, laugh for no reason or smack their lips.

Generalised tonic-clonic seizures: this is the best- known type of seizure. The whole body stiffens and shakes. Consciousness only comes back very slowly.

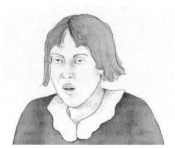 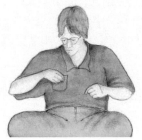

Abscence seizure   Complex partial seizure

Not every epileptic seizure is an emergency.

Seizures are not the fault of the teacher, the classmates or the school. They are part of a disorder. A seizure can rarely be stopped or prevented. If a seizure occurs, it is important to stay calm. Almost all seizures stop on their own.

At school children with epilepsy should be treated in the same way as other children.

What to do if a seizure occurs at school

- Stay calm, the seizure cannot be stopped.
- Make sure the child having the seizure is safe.
- Keep an eye on the time.
  Seizure should not last longer than 5-10 minutes.
- Observe the seizure and offer help after it has passed.

In status epilepticus an ambulance should be called.

In status epilepticus one seizure is followed by another. It is a medical emergency and has to be treated without delay. Status may just consist of two major seizures in one hour without full recovery of consciousness in between. In more severe status, major seizures may occur within minutes of each other.

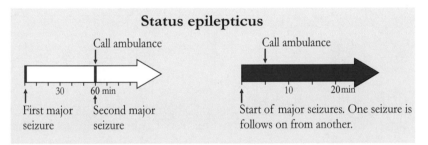

Status epilepticus

Call ambulance

30   60 min

First major   Second major
seizure   seizure

Call ambulance

10   20 min

Start of major seizures. One seizure is
follows on from another.

What **not** to do if a seizure occurs at school:

Panic - try to "wake up" the child having the seizure - try to stop the seizure - try to put antiepileptic drugs in the mouth - try to resuscitate during the seizure - put things in the mouth to stop people from "swallowing their tongue" - mouth to mouth breathing - hold the child down - leave the child alone - try to "wake up" the child from the sleep after the seizure.

Most seizures which happen at school are completely unpredictable. They may, however, be more likely with lack of sleep, stress, infections with high temperature, or on school trips.

Parents should tell teachers about their child's epilepsy

When teachers know that a child has epilepsy, they can try to help. Teachers will understand that a child's performance can vary if antiepileptic drugs have to be changed. Teachers can also try to make sure that a child with epilepsy is accepted by their classmates and does not feel excluded.

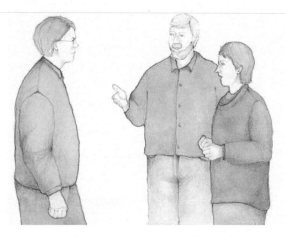

Children with epilepsy are normal children. Often, the only thing they know about their seizures is how people around them react to the attacks. Poorly-informed adults may react to seizures with fear or panic, which the children may not understand at all.

In some children, epileptic seizures are caused by other diseases, for instance disorders of the body's metabolism. Such children may have other problems as well as epilepsy.

Children who "only" have epilepsy can do just as well at school as other children.

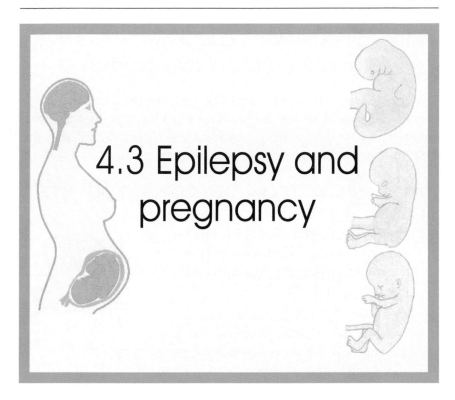

4.3 Epilepsy and pregnancy

Many people with epilepsy want to have a partner and to have children

Whether to marry or to have children are personal decisions which everybody should make for themselves. However, people with epilepsy may be able to avoid problems and reduce risks if they are well-informed about their condition and its treatment.

Things which may be considered when starting a family:

- Having a partner who also has epilepsy can improve mutual understanding. However, the risk of having children with epilepsy is higher if both parents have epilepsy.

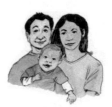

- It is important to tell a partner about epilepsy. A successful partnership is based on openness. This includes being honest about any health condition.

- Pregnancy should be planned well in advance. It is a good idea to think about childcare and how children will be looked after so that they will not be at risk of injury by their parents' seizures.

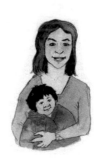

- Many antiepileptic drugs (like carbamazepine, phenytoin and topiramate) reduce the strength of the oral contraceptive pill; others do not (like valproate, lamotrigine, gabapentin and levetiracetam). Bleeding between periods is a sure sign that the oral contraceptive pill is not providing enough protection and other forms of contraception (like condoms) should be used.

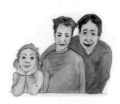

People with epilepsy have a slightly higher risk of having children with epilepsy

The size of the risk of having a child with epilepsy depends on the type of the father's or mother's epilepsy. On average the risk is around 3%. If both parents have epilepsy, the risk of children developing epilepsy is considerably higher.

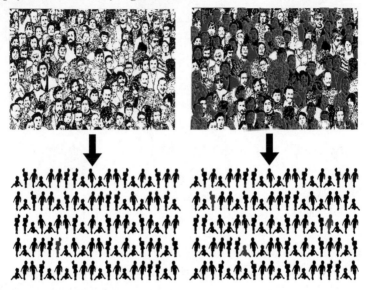

The picture gives an idea of the size of the risk. The left side shows that one out of 100 children born to parents without epilepsy will develop epilepsy. The right side shows what happens when one of the parents has epilepsy. Ninety-seven out of a hundred children will not have epilepsy.

If children born to parents with epilepsy develop epilepsy themselves, it is often the same type as their parents'. If, for instance, the father or mother developed absence seizures around the age of nine, it is most likely that the child (if they develop epilepsy) will also have absences. Epilepsy does not get worse by being passed on from parents to their children.

Antiepileptic drugs can damage babies in the womb

However, the risk of this is much lower than often thought.

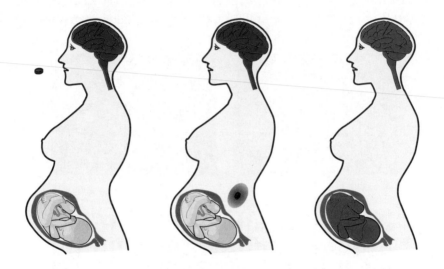

The drugs are taken up by the blood of the mother and taken to the brain. The baby in the womb is fed by the mother's blood. If antiepileptic drugs are carried by the blood, they can also reach the baby. All drugs have the potential to harm a baby in the womb. However, stopping antiepileptic drugs could cause a dangerous increase of the number of seizures or status epilepticus. This would be a serious risk to the health of the mother and, indirectly, to the health of the baby. During pregnancy the number of seizures can increase. However, some women also have fewer seizures. We do not fully understand how and why pregnancy can have different effects on epilepsy in different women.

Pregnancy causes a small increase of the risk of developing status epilepticus.

Mothers with epilepsy have a slightly higher risk of having children with abnormalities

Abnormalities are caused by problems with the development of the baby's body or organs. Examples of abnormalities include holes in the heart, or poor development of part of the face or the backbone.

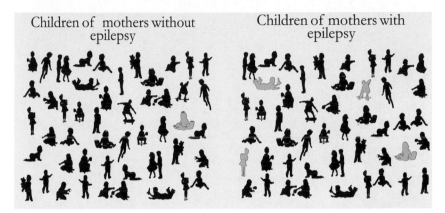

Children of mothers without epilepsy

Children of mothers with epilepsy

Parents without epilepsy can also have children with abnormalities.

The picture shows that one of 50 children born to mothers without epilepsy has an abnormality. Amongst mothers with epilepsy, abnormalities are found in four out of 50 children (shown on the right). These numbers include relatively small abnormalities like a slightly widened bridge of the nose. Severe abnormalities are less common.

Most abnormalities are caused by antiepileptic drugs. However, there is some evidence that seizures (especially status epilepticus) can also damage babies in the womb.

It can be dangerous to stop taking antiepileptic drugs out of concern about abnormalities! Medication changes are best discussed with a doctor.

The risk of abnormalities can be reduced if pregnancy is planned in advance

The baby's organs are formed in the first weeks and months of pregnancy. This is the time when abnormalities can develop.

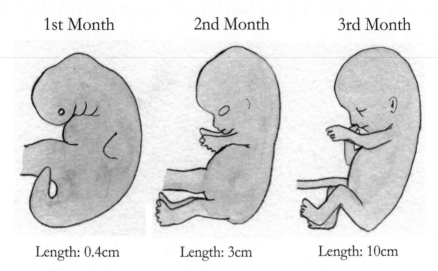

1st Month	2nd Month	3rd Month
Length: 0.4cm	Length: 3cm	Length: 10cm

It is best to talk to a doctor before conception to see how the risk of abnormalities can be reduced. There are a number of things which may be done:

- In certain cases, drugs may be withdrawn completely.
- Treatment may be changed from several drugs to one.
- It may be possible to lower the dose.
- It may be better to take several doses a day or switch to slow-release drugs.
- The diet may be improved to increase the intake of folic acid and other vitamins may be recommended.

Pregnancy should be planned well in advance.

Serious abnormalities can be discovered during pregnancy

Many serious problems with a baby's development can be picked up with an ultrasound examination. If a severe abnormality is found, further options can be discussed. In some cases, abnormalities can be treated with surgery once the baby has been born. In some cases, parents may think about having an abortion.

Severe abnormalities causing lifelong disability are very rare

Severe abnormalities often affect the heart, the brain or the spinal cord. Comparatively minor abnormalities (such as widely spaced eyes, a small nose which points upwards, short fingers and toes) are more common.

Most seizures do not affect the developing baby

A large number of major seizures (tonic-clonic) and status epilepticus are an exception. Status epilepticus can harm both mother and baby. There is no evidence that a single seizure affects the baby. It is not easy to weigh up the risks from antiepileptic drugs against the risks of having major seizures. It is best if this issue is discussed with an epilepsy specialist before pregnancy and if epilepsy is treated by a specialist during pregnancy.

Women with epilepsy can give birth in the normal way

Few women experience seizures during labour, although the risk of having a seizure is higher than usual around the time of delivery. It is important to try to take the antiepileptic drug in the usual way. Babies born to mothers taking certain antiepileptic drugs, which speed up the way the liver works, should be given an injection of vitamin K because there is a slightly higher risk of bleeding.

Antiepileptic drugs are also found in breast milk

Although antiepileptic drugs can be found in breast milk, the doses in the milk are usually so low that they do no harm to the baby. Breast milk also contains all the nourishment a baby needs and it strengthens the baby's defence system against infections. If the mother takes large doses of phenobarbital, primidone or benzodiazepines (for instance clobazam or clonazepam) as treatment for epilepsy, the drugs in the breast milk can cause babies to be sleepy and to suck poorly. If this happens, mothers can switch to bottle feeding altogether, or they can try a mixture of breast- and bottle- feeding.

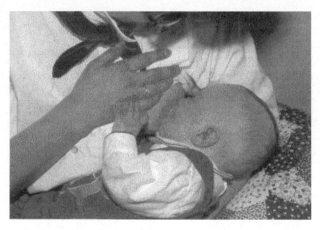

A child does not just bring joy but also stress and change. Often regular and sufficient sleep can only be guaranteed if both parents help, for instance when looking after the baby during the night. Breast milk can be pumped off so that the father can bottle-feed at night. If people have seizures which could put them at risk of dropping their baby, it may also be best for someone without epilepsy to bathe the baby.

Most women with epilepsy can breast-feed even if they are taking drugs to stop their seizures.

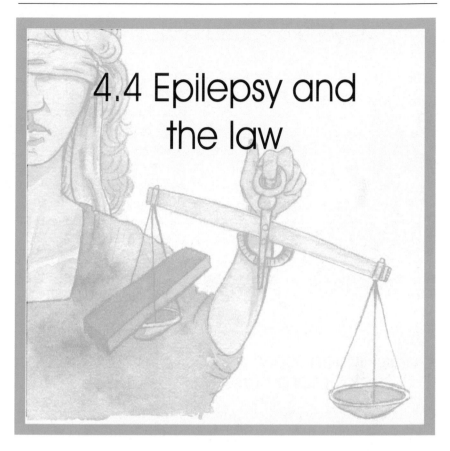

4.4 Epilepsy and the law

Everyone is equal before the law

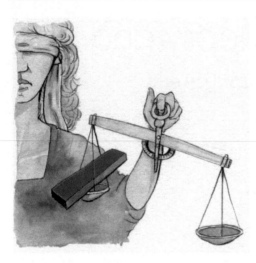

People with epilepsy must not face unfair discrimination because of their epilepsy. However, there are some situations in which people with epilepsy are not treated in the same way as others. People can only fight for their rights if they know what their rights are. Epilepsy can be an issue in legal disputes with employers or with insurance companies.

A child which "only" has epilepsy should go to a mainstream nursery and school.

Children with epilepsy without any additional learning disability or medical conditions have the same range of intelligence and abilities as children without epilepsy. Children with epilepsy and other conditions who need extra provision can have their needs met through Special Educational Needs legislation. For this reason, the majority of children with epilepsy are educated in mainstream schools or nurseries.

The Disability Discrimination Act covers children with epilepsy. This means that they have the same rights to attend the school of their choice as other children. Should a school refuse a child with epilepsy a place, this could be considered discriminatory. Unless there is absolutely no "reasonable adjustment" that the school could make to accommodate the child, the school's refusal of a place because of epilepsy would be against the law.

An epileptic seizure while driving a car can be very dangerous

To many people, driving is very important. The loss of a driving licence can cause considerable inconvenience. At the moment, the driving regulations say that people must have been free of all seizures for at least twelve months before they are allowed to drive an ordinary car. An exception is made for people who only ever have seizures during sleep: they may hold a driving licence (for a private car or motorbike) if there have been no attacks at all whilst they were awake for three years even if seizures during sleep continue. The driving regulations for heavy goods vehicles and for licences to transport passengers are much stricter. For a heavy goods licence for instance, people have to have been free of seizures and not taking antiepileptic drugs for ten years. More information is available from the DVLA Medical Unit, DVLA, Swansea, SA991TU, or from www.dvla.gov.uk.

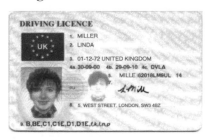
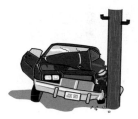

These regulations are not completely satisfactory because they do not take into account that seizures affect different people in different ways. Obviously it would be unsafe for someone to drive who has major seizures without warning. But what about people who only have attacks of twitching in one hand? They are banned because small seizures have the potential to develop into major seizures. But not all people with angina are banned from driving because they are at risk of heart attacks.

Very few accidents are caused by epileptic seizures.

People with epilepsy are only liable for damage caused by a seizure if they were "negligent"

It is very unusual that someone has to pay for damage caused by a seizure, although they could be held responsible if they had been negligent. As an example, someone with epilepsy may have to pay for damage caused during a seizure in a night club if they knew that the flashing lights would cause a seizure. Liability insurance may not have

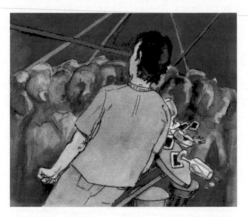

They would not have to pay for the damage if they had not known that flashing lights would trigger a seizure. Someone who has never had seizures before is not usually responsible for any damage

People with epilepsy are protected by the Disability Discrimination Act (1995)

Mr J. was offered a job as a clerical assistant. He agreed a start date and was then asked to have a health check. He revealed that he had epilepsy in the past but had not had any seizures since having epilepsy surgery. Within days of health check Mr J. was told that the vacancy was no longer available. When he took his case to an employment tribunal under the Disability Discrimination Act the company settled "out of court", paying Mr J. several thousand pounds in compensation.

Do employers have to be told about epilepsy?

There are very few jobs people with epilepsy are not allowed to do at all, for instance being an airline pilot or train driver. It is all right not to mention epilepsy at an interview for a job or on a job application form if an epileptic seizure in the work place would cause no more harm to yourself or to others than when at home or whilst out and about. This may be particularly appropriate if seizures have been fully controlled for months or years.

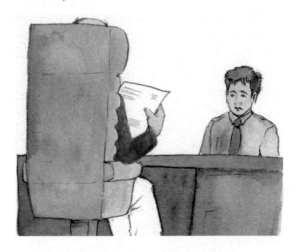

However, people have to be honest about epilepsy when they undergo a work-related medical check, for instance before they start a job. The Health and Safety at Work Act says that people also have to inform the employer about their epilepsy if their seizures could cause harm at a workplace. Depending on the seizure type and job, it may be possible to make the workplace safe. The employer, the union or the Employment Medical Advisory Service (EMAS) of the Health and Safety Executive may have ideas about how this can be done. If you decide to talk to an employer about epilepsy, it is best to be as matter-of-fact about your seizures as possible. It may be an idea to practice this in advance, for instance with friends or at the Jobcentre. You could also ask your doctor to write a letter about your epilepsy for your employer.

Insurance companies often want to know when epilepsy began

Insurance companies do not like risk. If an insurance company can prove that an illness or medical condition increases the risk that they may have to pay out, the premium will be higher or a policy may be refused altogether. Many insurance application forms ask about chronic illness or medical conditions. People who do not tell the truth on an application form may find that they have no cover if they try to submit a claim, even if they have paid their premiums on time. Some insurance policies also state that the person who has taken out the insurance has to inform the insurance company about changes in their health status. For instance, people who are first diagnosed with epilepsy may have to inform a private health insurance, motor or life insurance of their condition.

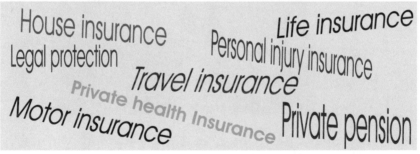

It can be difficult for people with epilepsy to get private health insurance. If epilepsy is diagnosed after health insurance has been taken out, the insurance company will not be able to increase the premium or refuse cover. Some insurance companies will try to exclude any claims caused by epilepsy. Sometimes such exclusions actually break the law. Self-help groups, disabled rights groups, the Citizens Advice Bureau or a lawyer may be able to help.

It can be a good idea to maintain insurance cover which was arranged before epilepsy was diagnosed.

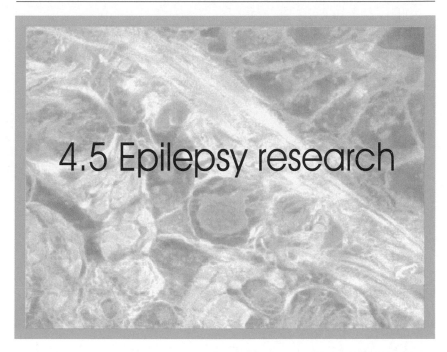

4.5 Epilepsy research

Knowledge about epilepsy has grown over many centuries

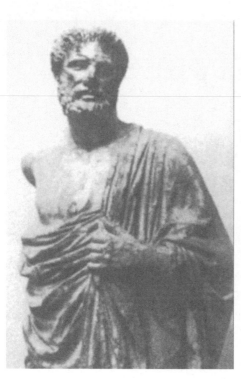

The word "epilepsy" was first used by Hippocrates over 2,000 years ago. Translated into English, it means something like "surprise attack". Hippocrates described epileptic seizures in a very detailed way, although his insights were forgotten in later centuries. It was often thought that people with epilepsy were possessed by demons or the devil. Treatment was often quite drastic. If treatment killed people, it was said that the demons were too strong. Some cultures also considered epilepsy a "sacred disease", thinking that people were close to God during a seizure.

Over many centuries epilepsy was a condition "one should not talk about". People with epilepsy were often excluded from public life. Because epilepsy was not discussed openly, most people knew very little about it. Lack of knowledge and prejudice made life hard for people with seizures. To some extent these problems still exist today - but we can try to change things. The history of the last 200 years shows how quickly knowledge about epilepsy can grow, but history also shows that such knowledge can be lost again.

Brain operations were performed in Egypt 3,000 years ago

The picture shows an operation performed about 500 years ago. This sort of surgery could have removed a blood clot from the brain. Such operations were very risky. Very few people would have survived.

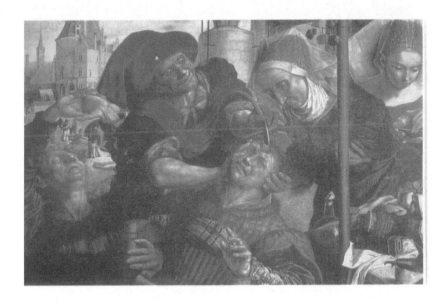

Today it is uncommon for someone to get worse rather than better through surgery. The risk of complications has become much smaller over the last 100 years. The main reason for this is the discovery that bacteria cause wound infection. This means that infections can be prevented. Great improvements have also been made in the field of anaesthesia so that it is now much safer to put people to sleep for operations. Modern medicine is the result of many small discoveries which have supported a process of continuous improvement. Of course, not every discovery leads to progress.

Epilepsy has been split into different types for over 100 years

Some types of epilepsy were first described by doctors who had someone with epilepsy in the family. This gave them the opportunity to observe the illness very closely.

James Edwin West had his first seizure in 1840 when he was four months old. He turned his eyes up and bent his head forwards, initially two to three times, later 50 to 60 times per day. Whereas only the head had been pulled up at first, it was soon the whole trunk. The head nearly touched the knees. Over the following years, James's physical development was normal but his mental development was slow. His father applied many different treatments. He tried bleeding, cold bandages, laxatives, opium and even poisons like hemlock. None of the treatments worked. At the age of three, the seizures decreased and James learned to stand.

James's father was a doctor who recorded his story in great detail. His description and treatment of James's illness was reported in medical journals and books. This means that James's type of epilepsy can now be recognised in other children. Today, it is called West syndrome. It remains a form of epilepsy which is difficult to treat.

In 1932 Hans Berger described the EEG as a new way of studying the brain

Initially Hans Berger hoped that he had found a method of investigation which would show what people thought. As it turned out, this was not possible. However, it was discovered that the EEG was a very useful investigation in the diagnosis and management of epilepsy. The EEG can be used to distinguish between different types of epilepsy and gives an idea where epilepsy comes from in the brain.

New methods of investigation increase our knowledge of how the brain works

The microscopes used over 100 years ago were good enough to show brain cells. This allowed the Spanish anatomist Ramon y Cajal to develop theories about the workings of the brain. Some of his ideas are still relevant today. Laser microscopes were developed about 30 years ago. They allow us to look at living tissue. The picture they produce is the result of complicated computer calculations.

The picture shows a a small piece of bowel wall. There are many muscle cells (shown in yellow). In the centre of the picture, there is a single nerve cell (shown in dark blue).

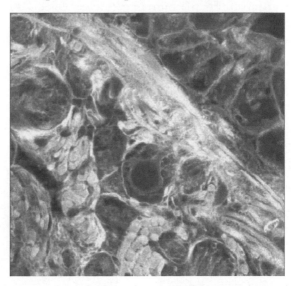

The invention of X-ray machines first made it possible to look inside the skull of living human beings. X-rays are invisible to the human eye. They pass through the body onto a photographic plate. The greater the density of the tissue they pass through, the fewer X-rays reach the plate. Bones are particularly dense. This means that it was not easy to make the brain visible with X-rays because it is surrounded by bone. It was not until 30 years ago that X-ray images of the brain could be produced with Computed Tomography (CT). A CT picture is the result of the computer analysis of X-rays passed through the skull from different directions.

Each nerve cell contains the blueprint of the body

This blueprint of the whole body is contained in the nucleus of each cell. It consists of a set of instructions, which can be read and carried out by the cells. These instructions are held on 46 chromosomes, which may be compared to books on a bookshelf. The books contain 50,000 different instructions (or genes). The instructions contained in the genes have been translated into a language which can be printed out on paper in the human genome project. It is likely that the results of this research will lead to advances in many fields of medicine, including the diagnosis and treatment of epilepsy.

The caterpillar and the butterfly have an identical set of genes. However, some genes are only switched on in the caterpillar, others only in the butterfly. Moreover, the same genes may have different effects depending on whether they are switched on in the caterpillar or the butterfly.

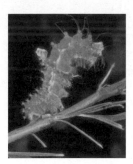 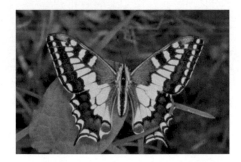

The translation of genes into the language of science can only explain a small (although perhaps important) part of how they work inside the body. One reason for this is that cells only read the instructions contained in a gene from time to time; another is that the same gene can have different effects in different cells of the body. The picture shows how complicated these things are. Using one set of genes, the same animal can live as a caterpillar or a butterfly.

Knowing the blueprint makes it possible to correct mistakes

It is likely that genetic tests will make it possible to diagnose epilepsy much more quickly, and to determine the type of epilepsy and the best treatment much more precisely in the future. Genetic tests for some rarer types of epilepsy are already available today. These are disorders in which epilepsy is caused by an error in the set of genetic instructions contained in the cell nucleus. Because all cells of the body carry the whole set of genetic instructions, such errors can be detected by blood tests. However, some people may have such an error in their genes without developing epilepsy.

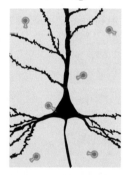

A nerve cell and viruses

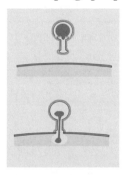

A virus injecting its genes (orange)

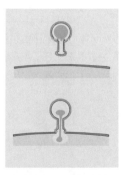

Viral genes replaced by a human gene (blue)

One particularly exciting branch of science is trying to develop tools which can be used to fix errors in the set of instructions held in the nucleus. Viruses are one such tool. Their own genes (which could damage the body's cells) can be removed and replaced by corrected human genes. The body's cells can then be infected with the virus, which would insert the correct instructions where they were needed. If the high hopes for this type of treatment become reality, medicine will change completely. There could be special viruses for countless diseases and many people with epilepsy could be cured. However, it may well take 100 years to get there.

New drugs have been developed

Seventy years ago there were few drugs which were effective against seizures. These included bromide, phenobarbital and phenytoin. About 30 years ago, a number of other antiepileptic drugs were developed. These were valproate, benzodiazepines, succinimides and carbamazepine. Over the last 10 years or so, further drugs have been added to the list of antiepileptic drugs available (oxcarbazepine, lamotrigine, vigabatrin, gabapentin, topiramate, tiagabine, zonisamide, levetiracetam and pregabalin). The modern drugs had to pass a lot of tests in animals and humans before they could be used by people with epilepsy.

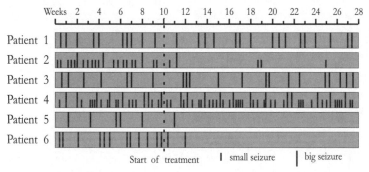

The picture shows seizure diaries covering 28 weeks. The seizures of six different people are recorded. Short red lines stand for minor seizures, long red lines for major seizures. Patient number one, for instance, only had major seizures about once per week. From week 10 onwards, patients received the tablets on trial. They continued to record their seizures.

Three patients were given tablets containing a new antiepileptic drug, and three received tablets which looked exactly the same but did not contain any medication. Neither the patients nor the doctors handing out the tablets knew who was taking medication and who was not. The picture shows that seizures in patients number two, five and six seemed to improve with the new treatment. After the study had been completed by all patients, it was checked whether these patients had received the new drug.

More new drugs are needed

One in four people with epilepsy cannot be treated successfully with the antiepileptic drugs available today. We do not fully understand why drugs do not stop seizures in some people. Do they have a type of epilepsy which is particularly difficult to control? Unfortunately, many of the new antiepileptic drugs are not "stronger" than the old ones. They work well in epilepsies which could also be treated with more established drugs, but their effects are disappointing in types of epilepsy which have proven hard to control.

In some ways, the discovery of new drugs is like fishing. The angler decides where he is going to throw the hook. But he is only guessing where the fish may be. He does not know for sure what is happening under the water surface. Sometimes he will be successful and catch a fish. At other times he will pull in an old boot or some weeds.

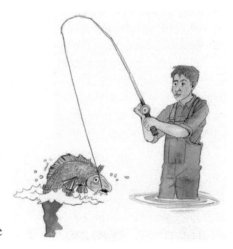

The development of new antiepileptic drugs is based on what is known about the chemistry of the brain. GABA, for instance, is a chemical messenger substance in the brain which is known to reduce activity in nerve cells. Increasing the effects of GABA could stop the development of epileptic activity in the brain. Given that GABA acts on the brain in this way, substances are being developed which could increase GABA activity. Once these substances can be made in the laboratory, their effect on epileptic seizures can be tested.

Tests on human brain cells can help

Operations are the treatment of choice for some problems of the brain, for instance for tumours. It is rarely possible to remove a tumour completely without cutting out some healthy brain tissue around it.

The removed tissue can be examined under the microscope after surgery. The examination of the tumour tissue determines the tumour type and is important for further treatment. Tests on the tissue around the tumour can help to find out how seizures start. However, such human brain tissue can only be used if the patient has given consent and agrees that some of the brain tissue removed at surgery can be used for research.

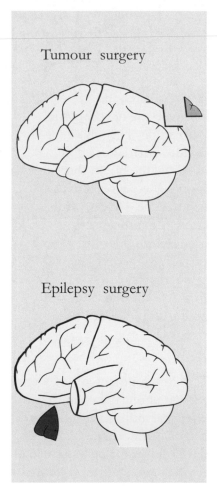

Tumour surgery

Epilepsy surgery

In operations for epilepsy, surgeons often have to remove a relatively large area of the brain to be sure that the whole epileptic area has been taken out. After surgery, the removed tissue is examined under the microscope for abnormalities. If they are preserved, brain cells can be kept "alive" for about ten hours. If patients have agreed that their brain tissue can be used for such tests, the tissue can be used to learn more about how seizures start.

Tests on animal brain cells are still necessary

Albino rats are used for many experiments intended to find out how epileptic seizures start or spread, and how they can be treated. For such tests, animals are anaesthetised and later put down.

Parts of the brain are removed and cut into thin slices. The brain cells in these slices can be kept "alive" for up to ten hours. The picture shows such a slice through the hippocampus. As in humans, seizures in rats often start in the hippocampus.

The brains of "lower" animals can also produce epileptic seizures. Some fruit flies (known as "shaker flies") can have seizures when they are exposed to ether. The picture shows a snail and nerve cells from the snail's brain. Some of the cells have been marked. The red cell can produce epileptic activity, the blue cell cannot. Now the differences between the two cells can be examined. Studying simple nervous systems like that of the snail can help to explain more complicated systems like human brains.

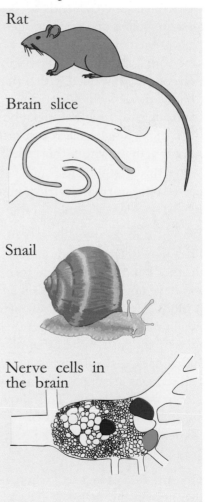

Rat

Brain slice

Snail

Nerve cells in the brain

Animals can also have epilepsy.

The workings of single nerve cells can be studied

To study electrical potentials in single cells, a thin glass tube is heated in the middle until the glass melts. When the two ends of the tube are pulled apart, the molten glass in the centre forms a very fine tube with a sharp tip. This micro-electrode is then filled with a fluid which conducts electricity. The electrode is so fine that it can be stuck into a single cell. It can record electric activity within this cell.

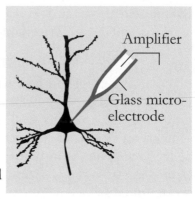

Using this method, it could be shown that epileptic seizures are caused by abnormal electric potentials in nerve cells of the brain.

The "patch-clamp"method is another important research tool. It was developed about 20 years ago. A blunt glass tube is pressed against a cell until its wall is stuck to the edge of the tube. When the tube is pulled back, a small part of the cell wall remains attached to it (as shown in the picture). This allows the study of the workings of channels within the severed part of the cell wall.

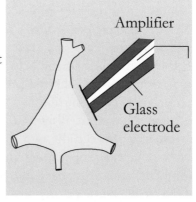

This method was used when it was discovered that the calcium channels in the cell wall let too much calcium into the cell when epileptic activity starts. In 1992 E. Neher and B. Sakmann received the Nobel prize for developing the "patch-clamp" technique.

It is still not known how exactly epileptic activity starts in the brain

We do not know what causes normal brain tissue to turn into tissue which can produce epileptic seizures. It has been sometimes observed that an epileptic focus in one half of the brain produces a so-called "mirror focus" on the opposite side, and that a mirror focus can then cause generalised seizures. It is, however, not known how this happens, and why it does not happen all the time.

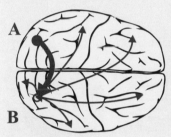

View of the brain from above

A: epileptic focus,
for instance due to a scar

➡ direction of first spread of epileptic activity.

B: "Mirror focus"

→ later spread and "generalisation" of epileptic activity.

The two halves of the brain are built in a very similar way. The right thumb, for instance, is moved by a particular area in the left half of the brain. Movements of the left thumb are controlled by the same area in the right half of the brain. Brain centres responsible for the same tasks of the right or left half of the body are closely linked by nerve fibres. Epileptic activity can spread through these connections, for example from the area in the left hemisphere which moves the right thumb to the area in the right hemisphere which moves the left thumb. This spread could cause a mirror focus. However it is not known how exactly this mirror focus develops.

Our knowledge about the start and spread of epileptic activity has many gaps. We can differentiate between a person's risk of having seizures, triggers for seizures and the suppression of seizures but we do not understand the mechanisms by which these processes happen.

More money needs to be spent on epilepsy research

There are many examples which show that science and medicine will advance if they are well-funded. More money would allow scientists to study a large range of important issues. For instance, there are some disorders of the body's metabolism which can cause epileptic seizures. Although the metabolic problems may be quite different, the seizures they cause look the same. It is likely that different metabolic disorders cause the same seizures in different ways. The diagram shows this more clearly.

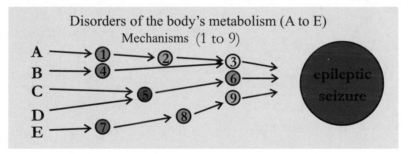

The disorders A to E lead to epileptic seizures through the mechanisms 1 to 9. We do not know what these mechanisms are. More research into this area could lead to the discovery of new ways of stopping seizures.

An epileptic focus could be treated like some tumours. Many tumours can be treated with particular types of poison. This form of treatment is called chemotherapy. The poison only affects the tumour and not the rest of the body, because it recognises some special feature which tumour cells do not share with healthy cells. It may be possible to find features of epileptic brain cells which they do not share with healthy brain cells. The epileptic cells could then be poisoned and destroyed in the same way as tumour cells are killed by chemotherapy. This could make it possible to cure people of epilepsy with a single course of treatment.

Sources:

M. Ebe, I. Homma: Leitfaden für die EEG-Praxis. Fischer, Stuttgart, 1992

C. Elger, A. Brockhaus, T. Grunwald: Epilepsie und Flugreisen. Dt. Univ.-Verlag, 1996

J. Engel, Jr., T.A. Pedley (Editors): Epilepsy. A comprehensive Textbook. Lippincott-Raven, Philadelphia, 1998

R.J. Gumnit: The Epilepsy Handbook. Raven, New York, 1995

H. Heintel: Quellen zur Geschichte der Epilepsie. Hans Huber, Bern, 1975

E.R. Kandel, J.H. Schwartz, T.M. Jessel: Principles of Neural Science. Raven, New York, 1996

A. Matthes: Epilepsien. Thieme, Stuttgart, 1984

K.L. Moore: Embryologie. Schattauer, Stuttgart, 1995

N.J. Pies: Biographisches und bibliographisches aus der Geschichte der Epilepsie. Robert Pfützner, München, 1990

D. Schmidt, C.E. Elger: Praktische Epilepsiebehandlung. Praxisorientierte Diagnose und Differentialdiagnose, rationale Therapiestrategien und handlungsorientierte Leitlinien. Thieme, Stuttgart, 1999

D.F. Smith, R.E. Appleton, J.M. MacKenzie, D.W. Chadwick: An Atlas of Epilepsy. The Parthenon Publishing Group Ltd., London, 1998

H. Stefan: Epilepsien Diagnose und Behandlung. In: Praktische Neurologie, B. Neundörfer, K. Schimrigk, D. Soyka (Hrsg.). VCH edition medizin, Weinheim, 1991

M.C. Walker, S.D. Shorvon: The British Medical Association Family Doctors Guide to Epilepsy. Dorling Kindersley, London, 1999

E. Wyllie (Hrsg.): The Treatment of Epilepsy. Lea and Febiger, Philadelphia, 1997

page 114: www.photocase.de (73402041196823HR)

Further reading

R. Appleton, B. Chappell, M. Beirne: Your child's epilepsy, a parents guide. Class Publishing, London, 1997. 240 pages.
Answers practical questions about epilepsy in children and how to live with it. Written for people looking after a child with epilepsy.

C.W. Bazil. Living well with epilepsy and other seizure disorders. Harper Resource, New York, 2004. 260 pages.
A detailed American paperback discussing many aspects of living with epilepsy and epilepsy treatment.

T. Betts, P. Crawford: Women and epilepsy. Martin Dunitz, London 1998. 84 pages.
Short summary of women's issues associated with epilepsy and treatment. Written for health professionals.

D. Chadwick (Editor): The encyclopedia of epilepsy. Roby Education Ltd., Merseyside, 1997. 60 pages.
Illustrated dictionary explaining epilepsy, its investigation and treatment to people with epilepsy.

A. Hanscomb, L. Hughes: Epilepsy (3rd Edition). Cassell Illustrated, London, 2002. 80 pages.
A short and illustrated book about epilepsy for people with epilepsy.

Useful addresses

Organisations for people with epilepsy in the UK and Ireland

Epilepsy Action
New Anstey House
Gate Way Drive
Yeadon
Leeds, LS19 7XY
Tel.: 0113/2108800
Freephone Helpline (UK):
0808/8005050
www.epilepsy.org.uk

National Society for
Epilepsy
Chasham Lane, chalfont St
Peter
Bucks. SL9 0RJ
Tel.: 01494/601300
www.epilepsynse.org.uk
Helpline: 01494 601 400

Brainwave - The Irish
Epilepsy Association
249 Crumlin Road
Dublin 12
Eire
Tel: +353 (0) 1/4557500
www.epilepsy.ie

Epilepsy Wales
15 Chester Street
St. Asaph
Denbigshire, LL17 0RE
Tel.: 01745 / 584444
Helpline: 08457/413774
www.epilepsy-wales.co.uk

Epilepsy Scotland
48 Govan Road
Glasgow G51 1JL
Tel.: 0141/4274911
Ftreephone Helpline:
0808 800 2200
www.epilepsyscotland.org.uk

Mersey Region Epilepsy
Association
The Glaxo Neurological
Centre
Norton Street
Liverpool, L3 8LR
Tel.: 0151/2982666
www.epilepsymersey.org.uk

Epilepsy Bereaved
PO Box 112
Wantage OX12 8XT
Tel.: 01235/772850
Bereavement contact line:
01235/772852
www.sudep.org.uk
*(Supports people bereaved through
an epilepsy-related death)*

Joint Epilepsy Council of the
UK and Ireland
Sharon Harvey
General Secretary
P.O. Box 186
Leeds, LS20 8WY
*(Information about voluntary
organisations for people with epilepsy)*

International epilepsy organisations

International Epilepsy
Resource Centre
IBE/ILAE
Swiss Epilepsy Centre
Bleulerstrasse 60
CH-8008 Zürich,
Switzerland
Tel.: +41 1/3876111
www.ierc.ch
*(Leaflets, pamphlets, guideline, CDs
and other information material
about epilepsy)*

Epilepsy Foundation (of
America)
4351 Garden City Drive
Landover, MD 20785 - 7223
Tel.: +1 / 800/3321000
www.efa.org

International Bureau for
Epilepsy
253 Crumlin Road
Dublin 12
Tel.: +353 1/4560298
www.ibe-epilepsy.org
*(Web links to epilepsy associations
throughout the world)*

International League Against
Epilepsy
Headquarters Office
Avenue Marcel Thiry 204
B-1200 Brussels
Belgium
Tel.: +32 (0) 2/7749547
www.ilae-epilepsy.org
*(Professional organisation for people
keen to improve epilepsy services)*

Epilepsy Association of
Australia
PO Box 879
Epping
Australia NSW 1710
Tel.: +61/1300/366162
www.epilepsy.org.au

Assessment, treatment, education and residential centres for people with epilepsy

National Society for
Epilepsy
Chasham Lane, chalfont St.
Peter
Bucks. SL9 0RJ
Tel.: 01494/601300
www.epilepsynse.org.uk
Helpline: 01494/601400

St Elizabeth's School
South End
Much Hadham
Hertfordshire, SG10 6EW
Te.: 01279/843451
www.stelizabeths.org.uk

Quarriers
Quarrier's Village
Bridge of Weir
Renfrewshire PA11 3SX
Tel.: 01505/616000 / 61224
www.quarriers.org.uk

The David Lewis Centre
Mill Lane
Warford nr. Alderley Edge
Cheshire, SK9 7UD
Tel.: 01565/640000
www.davidlewis.org.uk

The National Centre for
Young People with Epilepsy
St Pier´s Lane
Lingfield
Surrey, RH7 6PW
Tel.: 01342/832243
www.ncype.org.uk

Other useful organisations in the UK

Carers National Association
20-25 Glasshouse Yard
London EC1A 4JJ
Tel.: 0207/490888
www.londonhealth.co.uk/ca
rersnationalassociation.asp
carersline: 0345 573 369
(Advice on carers' rights)

DIAL UK
St Catherine's
Tickhill Road
Doncaster, DN4 8QN
Tel.: 01302/310123
www.dialuk.org.uk
(Advice on issues relating to disability)

Diasabled Living Foundation
380-384 Harrow Road
London, W9 2HU
Tel.: 0207/2896111
Helpline: 0845 130 9177
www.dlf.org.uk
*(Information on equipment to help
people with special needs)*

MENCAP (England)
123 Golden Lane
London, EC1Y 0RT
Tel.: 0207/4540454
www.mencap.org.uk
*(Advice and support for people
with learning disablilities)*

National Council for
Voluntary Organisations
(NCVO)
Regent´s Wharf
8 All Saints Street
London, N1 9RL
Tel.: 0207 7136161
www.ncvo.vol.org.uk
Helpline: 0800 2 798 798
*(Information about voluntary
organisations and charities)*

Patients Association
PO Box 935
Harrow
Middlesex, HA1 3YJ
Tel.: 0208/4239111
Helpline: 0845/6084455
www.patients-association.com
(Information about patients' rights)

Driving in the UK

Drivers Medical Group
DVLA
Swansea SA99 1DL
www.dvla.gov.uk
(Enquiries about driving licenses)

Holidays and sports for people with special needs

Holiday Care, Sunley House,
Croydon
4 Bedford Rd
Surrey, CRO 2AP
Tel.: 0845/124 9971
www.holidaycare.org.uk

BREAK
Davidson House
1 Montague Road
Sheringham
Norfolk, NR26 8WN
Tel.: 01263/822161
www.break-charity.org

RADAR (Royal Association for Disability and Rehabilitation) 12 City Forum 250 City Road London, EC1V 8AF Tel.: 0207/2503222 www.radar.org.uk	English Federation of Disability Sport Manchester Metropolitan University Alsager Campus, Hassall Road, Alsager Stoke-on-Trent, ST7 2HL Tel.: 0161/2475294 www.efds.co.uk

Identification bracelets or necklaces

Medic-Alert Foundation 1 Bridge Wharf 156 Caledonian Road London, N1 9UU Tel.: 0800/581420 www.medicalert.co.uk	SOS Talisman Talman Limited 21 Grays Corner Ley street Ilford, Essex Tel.: 0208 554 5579 www.sos-talisman.com

Medication aids (dosette boxes)

Chester Care Sidings Road PO Box 5665 Kirby-in Ashfield Notts., NG17 7QX Tel.: 01623/757955	Tempatron Ltd. 5 Darwin Close Reading Berks., RG2 0TB Tel.: 0118/9314062 www.tempatron.co.uk

Protection head gear

Aremco Grove House Old Ashford Rd. Lenham Kent, ME17 2PX Tel.: 01622/858502	Bradford Orthopaedic Services Ltd. Unit 3 Prince Valle Rd. Ind. Est. Duncombe Street Bradford, BD8 9AJ Tel.: 01274/481122

Seizure diary Year:

January

	6	12	18	hours
1				
2				
3				
4				
5				
6				
7				
8				
9				
10				
11				
12				
13				
14				
15				
16				
17				
18				
19				
20				
21				
22				
23				
24				
25				
26				
27				
28				
29				
30				
31				

February

	6	12	18	hours
1				
2				
3				
4				
5				
6				
7				
8				
9				
10				
11				
12				
13				
14				
15				
16				
17				
18				
19				
20				
21				
22				
23				
24				
25				
26				
27				
28				

March

	6	12	18	hours
1				
2				
3				
4				
5				
6				
7				
8				
9				
10				
11				
12				
13				
14				
15				
16				
17				
18				
19				
20				
21				
22				
23				
24				
25				
26				
27				
28				
29				
30				
31				

April

	6	12	18	hours
1				
2				
3				
4				
5				
6				
7				
8				
9				
10				
11				
12				
13				
14				
15				
16				
17				
18				
19				
20				
21				
22				
23				
24				
25				
26				
27				
28				
29				
30				

May

	6	12	18	hours
1				
2				
3				
4				
5				
6				
7				
8				
9				
10				
11				
12				
13				
14				
15				
16				
17				
18				
19				
20				
21				
22				
23				
24				
25				
26				
27				
28				
29				
30				
31				

June

	6	12	18	hours
1				
2				
3				
4				
5				
6				
7				
8				
9				
10				
11				
12				
13				
14				
15				
16				
17				
18				
19				
20				
21				
22				
23				
24				
25				
26				
27				
28				
29				
30				

July				August				September			
6	12	18	hours	6	12	18	hours	6	12	18	hours
1				1				1			
2				2				2			
3				3				3			
4				4				4			
5				5				5			
6				6				6			
7				7				7			
8				8				8			
9				9				9			
10				10				10			
11				11				11			
12				12				12			
13				13				13			
14				14				14			
15				15				15			
16				16				16			
17				17				17			
18				18				18			
19				19				19			
20				20				20			
21				21				21			
22				22				22			
23				23				23			
24				24				24			
25				25				25			
26				26				26			
27				27				27			
28				28				28			
29				29				29			
30				30				30			
31				31							

October				November				December			
6	12	18	hours	6	12	18	hours	6	12	18	hours
1				1				1			
2				2				2			
3				3				3			
4				4				4			
5				5				5			
6				6				6			
7				7				7			
8				8				8			
9				9				9			
10				10				10			
11				11				11			
12				12				12			
13				13				13			
14				14				14			
15				15				15			
16				16				16			
17				17				17			
18				18				18			
19				19				19			
20				20				20			
21				21				21			
22				22				22			
23				23				23			
24				24				24			
25				25				25			
26				26				26			
27				27				27			
28				28				28			
29				29				29			
30				30				30			
31								31			

Short dictionary of medical words

Absence: Epileptic seizure with brief blackout but no convulsion

Action potential: Electric signal used by the brain to pass on information from cell to cell

AED: Commonly used abbreviation for anti-epileptic or anticonvulsant drug

Allergic reaction: Reaction caused by being oversensitive to certain drugs mostly affecting the skin (red spots)

Ambulatory EEG: Prolonged EEG recording with a portable machine similar to a walkman

Amygdala: Part of the limbic system in the temporal lobe

Angiography: Method of showing up blood vessels using X-rays

Ataxia: Clumsiness, difficulty with coordination of movement, staggering walk. Common side-effect of antiepileptic drugs

Aura: The same as a small seizure (simple partial seizure), warning before more major seizure

Benign: Likely to take a good course, to respond to treatment, not to get worse, opposite of malignant

Biofeedback: Method of making the unconscious workings of the brain visible to teach people to influence them

Brain scan: Painless and harmless method of taking pictures of the brain, either using x-rays (computed tomography, CT) or radio waves (magnetic resonance imaging, MRI)

Callosotomy: Operation in which the connecting wires between the left and right half of the brain are cut

Catamenial epilepsy: Epilepsy with seizures occurring during menstruation

Cerebral hemispheres: The two halves of the cerebrum (brain). The left hemisphere controls the right half of the body, the right hemispere the left half

Cerebrospinal fluid (CSF): Fluid which surrounds the brain and is not in direct contact with the blood

Cerebrum: Major part of the brain controlling all conscious brain functions

Clonic seizure: Seizure with brief muscle twitching

Cluster: A number of seizures close together

Complex partial seizure: Partial seizure with impairment of consciousness

Compliance: Taking tablets as they were prescribed

Convulsion: Latin name for seizure

Computed Tomography (CT): Method of showing the shape and the structures of the brain using X-rays and computers

Corpus callosum: Bundle of wires connecting the right and left half of the brain

Cryptogenic epilepsy: Type of focal epilepsy in which the site of the focus cannot be found

Cyanosis: Blue colouring of the skin. Sign of low oxygen in the blood. May occur during generalised convulsions

Déjà vu: French for "seen before". Feeling of unusual familiarity

Desensitisation: Method of reducing the sensitivity to certain physical or mental processes to reduce their effects on the body

Developmental delay: Slower than expected course of a child´s usual development

Differential diagnosis: Range of medical explanations for a symptom. Loss of consciousness can be caused by epilepsy, fainting, psychogenic seizures etc.

Dossette box: Box for a one-week-supply of medication with several compartments for drugs for each day. Helps people to remember to take their tablets regularly

EEG: Electroencephalogram. Method of studying the electric function of nerve cells in the brain

Encephalitis: Infection or inflammation of the brain. May cause epilepsy

Epilepsia partialis continua: Condition in which one partial seizure is immediately followed by another

Epilepsy specialist nurse: Nurse who has undergone special training to advise people with epilepsy

Febrile convulsions: Seizures in small children triggered by high temperatures

Focal seizure: Seizure starting from one small area (focus) of the brain. Identical to "partial seizure"

Focus: area of the brain which is able to produce epileptic activity

Frontal lobe: The front part of each hemisphere of the brain

Generalised seizure: A seizure with epileptic activity in both halves of the brain

Generic name: Name of the chemical substance used in an antiepileptic drug.

Grand-mal seizure: Major seizure consisting of a period of stiffening (tonic phase) and a period of jerking (clonic phase)

Hemispherectomy: Removal of part of the brain to stop seizures. May be performed after brain inflammation, infection or injury in children

Hippocampus: Part of the temporal lobe involved in transferring memories from short to long-term stores. Frequently source of seizures

Hypermotor seizure: Seizure causing wild and uncontrollable movements of the body starting in the frontal lobes, often from sleep

Hyperventilation: Increased breathing without increased activity, overbreathing

Ictal: During an epileptic seizure

Idiopathic generalised epilepsy: Epilepsy of unknown cause and place of seizure onset in the brain with involvement of both halves of the brain from the beginning of a seizure

Interictal: In between seizures

Intramuscular: Into a muscle

Intravenous: Into a vein

Jacksonian seizure: Seizure in which movements or sensations spread over one side of the body

Ketogenic diet: Consists of protein and fat and can reduce seizures after some days

Lesion: Area of damage or disease in the body

Limbic system: Parts of the brain important for feelings

Lobes: Parts of the cerebral hemispheres

Magnetic Resonance Imaging (MRI, also known as **MR Tomography, MRT)**: Method of producing pictures of the living brain using radio waves

Metabolism: The making and breakdown of substances in the body

Myoclonus: Brief muscle jerk

Occipital lobe: Back part of both hemispheres of the brain

Oral: By mouth

Parietal lobe: Part of both hemispheres below the crown of the skull

Partial seizure: Epileptic seizure involving only a part of the brain (identical to focal seizure)

Photosensitivity: Ability of the brain to react to flashing lights by producing epileptic activity

Positron Emission Tomography (PET): Method of producing pictures of the metabolism of the brain

Postictal: Immediately after a seizure

Prognosis: Outlook, likely future development

Provocation: Method of triggering a seizure

Provoked seizures: Seizures which did not happen spontaneously but had a clear cause like a head injury or stroke

Psychogenic seizure (also known as non-epileptic functional or pseudoseizure): Seizure which looks like an epileptic seizure but is not caused by electric discharges in the brain

Rectal: Through the back passage

Retard-preparation: Form of

tablets which ensures that drugs are only released slowly from the bowel and work longer

Rolandic epilepsy: Benign form of epilepsy starting in the frontal lobe

Sapphire Nurse: Epilepsy specialist nurse provided through funding from Epilepsy Action

Secondary generalisation: Seizure spreading from one part to the rest of the brain

Seizure diary: Diary in which seizures and possible triggers are recorded to observe the course of epilepsy

Seizure threshold: Likelihood of developing seizures. People with a low threshold are at greater risk of having seizures

Sleep deprivation: Method of causing lack of sleep to try to provoke seizures in hospital

SPECT scan (short for Single Photon Emission Computed Tomography): Type of a scan which can help to find the source of epileptic seizures

Spike and wave pattern: EEG appearance typically found in people with epilepsy

Status epilepticus: Condition in which one seizure is followed by another without recovery in between, medical emergency

Syndrome: Combination of features of a particular illness found in many people, type of illness

Remission: Improvement of illness, when epileptic seizures stop

Temporal lobe: Part of the brain behind the temple

Todd's paralysis: Weakness of one side of the body immediately after a seizure

Tonic-clonic seizure: Also known as grand-mal. Generalised seizure with stiffening followed by shaking

Tonic seizure: Seizure with brief stiffening of the body

Trigger factor: An event which usually starts off a seizure

Vagal nerve stimulator: Electric stimulator similar to a pacemaker which reduces seizures by sending electric impulses along the vagal nerve

Videotelemetry: Recording seizures with video and EEG

Index

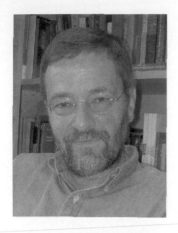

Ulrich Altrup is Professor of Medicine at the Faculty of Medicine, University of Münster, Germany. He holds the chair of Experimental Epileptology and has a scientific interest in the mechanisms causing epileptic activity in the brain. He trained in the fields of Physiology and Epileptology and he is engaged in public education on medical topics.

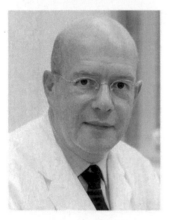

Christian Elger is Professor of Epileptology at the University of Bonn, Germany. He is the head of one of the most important epilepsy surgery and epilepsy research centres in Europe. Much of his research and his work for organisations like the International League against Epilepsy has helped to reduce the stigma associated with epilepsy.

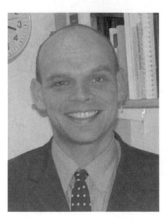

Markus Reuber is a Senior Lecturer and Consultant Neurologist in Sheffield, UK. His research has concentrated on how to diagnose and treat seizure disorders. He has a particular interest in improving communication between doctors and people with epilepsy and is a member of the Council of Epilepsy Action.